Feeding
your
Children

Feeding
your
Children

A complete guide to healthy eating for pregnancy, babies, toddlers and children up to 11

Miranda Hall

PIATKUS

© 1984 Miranda Hall

First published in 1984 by Judy Piatkus (Publishers)
Limited of London

Reprinted 1986, with amendments

British Library Cataloguing in Publication Data
Hall, Miranda
    Feeding your children.
    1. Children – Nutrition
    I. Title
    613.2′088054   RJ206

        ISBN 0–86188–266–0 (hardback)
        ISBN 0–86188–319–5 (paperback)

Edited by Susan Fleming
Designed by Dave Allen
Drawings by Margaret Leaman

Typeset by Phoenix Photosetting, Chatham
Printed and bound by Garden City Press. Letchworth

To my sons Simon and Robin
(who were such a challenge, and in their early years so often tried my patience!)
and to my husband Peter
(who never lost his).

Contents

Acknowledgements

I should like to acknowledge the help and encouragement I have always received from Mary Berry since our teenagers were toddlers. It was Mary who urged me to record for others what I had discovered in my research into feeding both babies and children.

This is an age when many powerful bodies have as yet largely ducked the responsibility of providing us with the food we *need*, and the information and education to choose it wisely to ensure the better health of our children. Departments of Agriculture, Fisheries and Food, Ministries of Education and of Health, and our food industry have all avoided the problem as a whole, and blame each other for not guaranteeing the better health of our young families. Yet it is very refreshing to find people who *do* care, who *do* want to protect the health of our children, who will bring new findings to our attention, who will help us as individual parents, and who will organise and fund research. So that others may seek their help too, their addresses are at the end of this book. I am most grateful to them for the information they have given, and for their continued search to ensure our children have a better and healthier future.

Introduction

Few of us can be unaware of the importance that is now being attached to the value of a healthy diet. While many only come to terms with the essentials of good nutrition long after they have *left* childhood, it is increasingly clear to nutritionalists that health can be much altered by the diet *in* childhood, and *before* childhood. In fact, even *before* conception the good diet of both parents is now seen as vital to ensure the foetus may have the very best possible start in life. It is amazing to me that while sheep farmers and other animal breeders are conscious of this fact, men and women – often carefully planning their families in other respects – seem to remain ignorant of the importance of this preparation (sometimes through lack of interest, often through lack of relevant information and education).

Good nutritious food is vital throughout life, but especially just before and during pregnancy, and through childhood in this age of 'fast', processed, over-refined, and 'junk' food. Before many mothers are aware they are pregnant, in the first weeks of the embryo's development, the limbs and organs of their baby are being formed; this new active life needs proper nutrients from its mother's diet for growth and can be damaged by mal-nutrition, smoking, alcohol or drugs. And later, weaning a baby is too important to be left to chance; as research into allergies has shown, much long-term damage is linked to many basic foods an ill-informed mother may give her baby in his or her early months. Every parent needs up-to-date information on how to choose the optimum diet, at each stage, to ensure the proper mental and physical development and growth of their child.

Only to list foods you *should not* give to your babies or children is just too dreary and depressing. What mothers need to know is which foods they *can* give their children which will be enjoyed, and how to tempt those faddy toddlers and yet do so with the confidence of having chosen foods which will supply their real needs. Worried parents need the comfort and reassurance that they are offering suitable foods and drinks when their children are ill, or when they refuse to eat breakfast or school lunches.

After extensive training in cookery, both as a science and as an art, I innocently believed feeding my family would present few difficulties. Yet when I was actually faced with all the problems every parent encounters, I realized how ill-equipped I was, and how pitifully ill-informed most young mothers were. Because my own children proved such a challenge, and showed up my weaknesses, I determined to find some answers.

Every parent wants to give their children the best care in every possible way, and wants to know which are the best foods. Commercial food companies and their advertisers continually persuade us which foods to eat: they beguile parent and child alike, informing us of some small value their products have, but not warning us of what nutrients their products have lost, nor of how their food additives may affect the mental and physical health of our children. These foods are often eaten in quantity at the expense of the real foods young bodies need, and many childhood ailments and tantrums can be directly attributed to them.

Food should be a pleasure to prepare, cook and eat, especially when you can do it all with confidence. Many parents need only to adjust their diet a little in order to eat well and wisely, but children are perhaps the worst-fed members of our society; little thought is given to the quantity of junk food they eat or what they eat when at school; children are given no information on even the basics of nutrition until they are about fourteen, and yet most are allowed to choose their food freely. These children are supposed to be our hopes for a new and healthier generation, yet are taking with them into adult life a terrible legacy of rotten teeth, premature heart disease, unnecessary allergies, overweight, poor eating habits, and sometimes, sadly, mental and physical handicap.

This book is the outcome of many years' research. Its aim is to inform parents and give them the courage to choose food wisely, well and with enjoyment to ensure the health and happiness of their children. It is full of information on every aspect of infant and child feeding, but it also contains some uncompromising advice and warnings that may alarm some parents. It is based on facts from our present knowledge of nutrition, from medically researched recommendations, from information from food manufacturers, and from my own personal experience, not only as a teacher and writer on infant feeding, but also as a mother.

The facts in this book could be regarded as the building blocks for a new healthier generation. A good diet should be a way of life for every parent and child, and it is never too early – or too late – to learn to eat well and wisely, and I hope that this book may help.

Miranda Hall
February 1984

Chapter One
Good nutrition for all

Understanding the basic facts about nutrition will help you to choose a better diet for yourself, and for your family. There are two primary stages of growth in the life of a child when the calorie requirements are low but the nutritional demands are very high. The first is while the child is still in the womb, and the second is during the first three years of life. No amount of good food later in life can make up for deficiencies in these periods of development and growth. It is essential, therefore, to understand the value of different foods in order to serve a balanced selection to your family – foods which contain adequate proteins, carbohydrates, fats, vitamins and minerals, all the essentials of good health.

From the start it is important to plan your child's diet. Great care must be taken when moving to solid feeding, and there must not be a slide in the pre-school child's diet to the wide use of 'foods' with little or no value. Between the ages of five and eleven years steer your child into making a sensible choice of food. By eleven, children will have much greater freedom in the spending of pocket money, and in the choice of school lunch if it is a help-yourself canteen service. Your influence then will be minimal. Up to this stage, you have been responsible for choosing the foods your children should eat, and you can have omitted any you thought were unsuitable. Although you cannot *make* children eat what you think they should, you can reduce the problem by not having unsuitable foods around, and children are likely to eat what is suitable – what you *do* have available – from pure hunger.

The diet of many in the more affluent societies is adequate, often *too* adequate, in quantity, but very inadequate in quality. Food with high nutritional value is not necessarily more expensive – indeed it is sometimes considerably *less* expensive. It is easy to find good food in the average high street or super-market. And by good food, I mean fresh foods mainly: fresh meat, fresh fish, fresh vegetables, fresh fruit. Much of this good food is not expensively refined or manufactured and, as a result, it does not create the need for heavy advertising to tempt the ill-informed public.

It is undoubtedly true that manufacturers of food products have two major duties: to keep its work-force in business, and to make a profit for its share-holders or owners. By law, their produce must be hygienic and not toxic, and by law some limitations are put on the contents they may use and the descriptions given to their products. *But*, they are under no obligation to provide a healthy, well-balanced diet; they are not required to provide what the public need or should eat – only what they *will* and *do* eat, which is a very different matter. Many of the products from the manufacturing food industry can be termed 'junk food'. They contain calories to satisfy our need for energy but may completely lack proteins, vitamins, minerals and fibre. They are very high in chemical additives such as preservatives, stabilisers etc., and are often highly coloured and flavoured to deceive the eye and taste buds.

The food you buy

Ideally the greatest part of the diet – for children *and* for adults – should be of the freshest fruit, vegetables, fish and lean meats plus grains, with the minimum of refinements. In the following pages are listed the basic nutritional elements required by the body from food, and in the chapters thereafter ways of using those elements to the fullest possible health advantage. Once aware of the life-long value of good nutrition, you will never again eat or drink something without being aware of what good – or bad – it is doing you (and the listing at the end of this chapter of the diseases that can be caused by bad diet or dietary deficiencies is *horrifying*).

Although fresh is undoubtedly best, in practice most of us have to rely on what our local supermarkets offer, and convenience plays an important part in the foods we choose.

Convenience foods

When buying processed foods always look carefully at the labels for the list of contents. Aim at goods low in the following: sugar, starch, modified starch, nitrates, salt, sodium, monosodium-glutamate, emulsifiers, preservatives, colouring, flavourings and vaguely termed edible fat. These are always listed in descending order of quantity.

Breakfast cereal details are given in Chapter Six to help you get the best value in regard to nutrition and economy. Remember that unrefined cereals such as muesli contain extra valuable nutrients not listed, particularly if made from natural unheated grains, nuts and fruits. Many of the muesli-type breakfast cereals are *toasted* grains or very high in sugar.

Frozen foods

Simple frozen foods such as fruit, vegetables, meat and fish without coatings and pastry etc., are always a good choice if fresh is not readily available. They will have lost only a little in nutritional value. From January to May vegetables, especially home-frozen, will provide a wide variety, and costs can compare favourably with much fresh produce during this season. Poultry, meat and fish will compare well in food value with fresh products; poultry and some meat will in fact be cheaper bought frozen. There is some loss of flavour in frozen goods. Products made from meat and fish should need far fewer preservatives than other packaged goods which is an advantage. Those pies, pastries, pizzas, rissoles, burgers and other processed products need labels checked very carefully for contents so that you are giving the family the ingredients they need. Fish fingers usually contain 50 per cent fish; the larger they are the less coating to fish, so buy larger ones or coat fish yourself with nutritious chemical-free coatings. In products of which pastry is a major part, you will be paying a high price for the small proportion of ingredients which are nutritionally of some real value. On the whole most processed prepared frozen products (pies, cakes, pastries, ice cream, pizzas, lasagne, burgers etc.) are high in animal fat, salt or sugar and refined starches, and low in protein, fibre, vitamins and minerals. Although convenient these more processed products should never be used as a major part of the diet.

Tinned and vacuum jar foods

All list contents in descending order to make an objective choice easier. Tomatoes and fruits canned in their own juice will only lose Vitamin C but retain other vitamins and minerals without unnecessary sugar and starch; colour, flavour and other chemicals will normally not be added. Tinned sweetened fruit and pie fillings provide much less fruit than you might imagine; only a few carry details of weight of minimum fruit content which is the important constituent, and may be very high in sugar and modified starches.

Tinned fish is usually good value. Mackerel and sardines are often preferred by children packed in tomato juice instead of oil or brine. Tinned meats need careful examination so that you buy what you expect; some are very deceptive in the meat content.

Tinned and packet soups are of very poor nutritional value, so do not give value for money when considering family housekeeping. They give calories and the impression that food has been eaten but in reality provide little goodness. With a processor or blender, fresh or left-over cooked vegetables and casseroles etc. which might otherwise be thrown away, can be quickly turned into nutritious soups, diluted with milk or stock at a negligible cost, and take only a few minutes to prepare.

Tinned beans must be graded a first-class convenience food. They provide very useful protein, vitamins, minerals and fibre and a minimum of fat which far outweighs the content of sugar, salt and refined starch. They contain no preservatives, colour or artificial flavour. Choose those brands that contain most beans to sauce, not the cheapest. The extra few pence for this cheap food are worth it. Similar convenience foods, like tinned spaghetti in tomato sauce, are inferior in food value as they lack the fibre and quality of proteins, minerals and vitamins which the beans provide.

Dried foods

Dried fruit is a very useful addition to a child's diet. High in potassium for the release of energy plus other minerals, they are a good balancing ingredient for those taking too much salt. Much better than sweets for a quick snack. Currants, raisins and sultanas are good, and do remember mixed dried apricots, peaches, apples, pears, dates and prunes. Health-food shops will stock bananas, figs, pawpaw, pineapple and other exotic dried fruits as an alternative. The less sticky make the most portable snacks, and they are ideal for packed lunches or break-time. Dried fruits should not be considered a source of Vitamin C, and should be sun-dried for preference (the commercial method of drying in ovens with sulphur dioxide can create a kidney irritant if eaten in large quantities).

Many packaged dried fruit – raisins and sultanas, for instance – have mineral oil added to prevent fruit drying excessively or sticking. Mineral oil is a laxative and draws fat-soluble vitamins (A, D, E, and K) from the body. Choose brands that do not contain oil or rinse fruit under warm water quickly, especially for small children.

Dried vegetables like peas, beans, lentils and other seeds, are a rich source of protein, B vitamins, minerals and fibre, an excellent addition to the diet. Freeze-dried onions, peppers, peas and green beans are of less nutritional value than frozen or fresh, but may be useful occasionally. They will not provide Vitamin C.

Dried pasta adds some protein and other nutrients to the diet, and wholemeal pasta is particularly nutritious. Pot noodles and similar products to which boiling water is added are of very little nutritional value. They should not be used as an alternative to a proper meal, being low in protein, fibre, minerals and vitamins and very high in chemical additives.

Other dried goods have large areas of supermarkets devoted to them, and they cannot be considered 'foods', particularly for young children with smallish appetites. Crisps and similar items – biscuits, instant puddings, convenience puddings, instant and other drinks – should all be considered carefully before purchase to decide whether they will really contribute to your family's diet and health. Once you purchase many of these items they will be eaten in preference to nutritious foods, and will lead to pressure from your family to constantly supply them.

Calories

Calories – the means by which the energy value of food is measured – are present in all foods, and a certain proportion are necessary each day for all of us, to maintain growth and good health. In a baby, most calorie requirements will be supplied by milk.

To convert calories to use for energy our bodies use protein, B vitamins and minerals. Fats, sugars and refined starches provide none of these yet by consuming them they deplete our body's stores. To

Recommended Daily Calorie Requirements	
Under 1 year	800
1–2 years	1,200–1,400
3–4 years	1,600
5–6 years	1,800
7–8 years	2,100
9–11 years	2,300–2,500
Teenage	2,300–3,000
Mothers	2,300
Expectant mothers	2,400
Lactating mothers	2,700
Fathers	2,700–3,600

maintain good health we should severely limit intake of these foods.

The calorie needs of individuals vary considerably; the above chart is only a guide to a recommended daily calorie intake.

Proteins

These are required by the body for growth and repair of all the organs of the body: heart, lungs, liver and kidneys. They are needed by the brain and nervous system, and by the muscles and skin, by the glands, hormones and enzymes of the body. During pregnancy, infancy, childhood and adolescence – all the times of major growth – the need for protein is at its greatest. Insufficient may cause deterioration in mental and physical health, and in pregnancy and infancy, severe deficiency can arrest the mental development of the child.

Those most at risk of having too little for their needs are expectant mothers, infants and young children eating a poor diet, particularly those who start too early mixed feeding. Some elderly people are also on too low a protein diet. Conversely, many adults are now considered to be on too high a protein diet for good health. Having too much protein can damage the health as easily as having too little. Surplus protein that we do not need for repair or growth of the body is either converted to use for energy, or is deposited as fat, which is downright dangerous. Those eating large cooked breakfasts, massive steaks or other meats at midday and in the evening, and who lead a sedentary life-style, are all eating and living badly. It is a diet favoured by many men – particularly those enjoying expense-account lunches – and can lead to premature diseases of old age, as well as overweight.

Recommended Daily Protein Requirements	
Under 1 year	¾ oz (20 g)
1–2 years	just over 1 oz (30–35 g)
3–4 years	1¼ oz (40 g)
5–6 years	1½ oz (45 g)
7–8 years	1¾ oz (55 g)
9–11 years	just over 2 oz (65 g)
Teenage	2¼–2½ oz (70–75 g)
Mothers	1¾–2 oz (55–65 g)
Expectant mothers	about 2 oz (60–65 g)
Lactating mothers	2–2¼ oz (68–70 g)
Fathers	2–3 oz (65–90 g)

(Men or women with very active occupations have a greater need for protein for the repair of worn and damaged body cells.)

Approximately ¼ oz (7 g) protein is provided by each of the following:

1 cup milk
1 oz (30 g) meat, fish, bacon, chicken
1 oz (30 g) cheese (Cheddar type)
1 small carton yogurt
2 oz (60 g) oatmeal
2 oz (60 g) dry pasta
2 oz (60 g) wholemeal bread
2 tablespoons wheatgerm
2 tablespoons peanut butter
2 oz (60 g) sausage
2 Shredded Wheat
4 oz (115 g) peas
5 oz (150 g) baked beans

Animal and vegetable proteins

Proteins were formerly divided into two groups: those which provide a complete range of amino acids and those which supply a limited range only. Amino acids are the basic constituents of protein, and there are over twenty, many of which the body can convert one to another, according to its needs. Some, however, the body cannot synthesise, and they must be provided adequately in the diet. Those foods that contain all the amino acids we cannot convert ourselves, but need, were called *complete proteins*. These are supplied by the following foods:

Milk (human, animal, and dried)
Meat and poultry, fish, eggs
Cheese and yogurt
Soya beans (the only food of non-animal origin which is a complete protein).

Remaining protein foods which do not contain all the essential amino acids were known as *incomplete proteins*. They remain a most useful source of protein, and are usually much cheaper than the animal proteins. They are:

Grains especially whole grains and wheatgerm, wheat, oats, rye, rice, etc., and all produce made from them – pasta, bread, breakfast cereal
Pulses all dried beans, lentils, peas, beans and bean sprouts
Nuts and seeds including peanut butter, sesame seeds, sprouted seeds etc.

By combining complete proteins with incomplete proteins, or grains with pulses and nuts, we use these highly nutritious foods with greater efficiency and considerably less cost. For example, milk with cereals; macaroni cheese; egg sandwich; spaghetti bolognese; muesli and pizza. These relatively inexpensive foods can provide as much useful protein as expensive steaks and chops.

Fat

Those fats we are most aware of consuming are butter, oil, margarine, lard, dripping and fat on meat. In our diet, we consume in total quite a large quantity from less visible sources – in milk, cheese, nuts, in lean meat and oily fish, offal, egg yolk, vegetables and seeds. There are particularly large quantities of fats in pastry, pies, sausages, pâté, luncheon meats, cakes, biscuits and prepared foods.

Some types of fat or oil are essential for the good healthy working of the body. They are mainly polyunsaturated fats and are found in seeds, grains and vegetable oils. Only very small quantities of these fats are needed – about 1 to 2 per cent of the energy intake of the body. These polyunsaturated fats – low in cholesterol – are oils at room temperature but are hardened to make soft margarines like Flora and sunflower. These spreading fats have additional advantages, in that being very soft, they can be spready more thinly and are quick to use in baking. Fats that are not of this type, the saturated fats, contribute to the cholesterol level in the blood vessels. Although adults should be careful in their consumption of *all* fats, a *moderate* amount is necessary for a baby and growing child.

Fats and oils play two other major roles in our diet: they are responsible for the absorption of the fat-soluble Vitamins A, D, E and K; they also considerably add to our enjoyment of food, making it more palatable and tasty, adding rich flavour to casseroles, sauces etc. It is very important that food is enjoyed, one of the great pleasures of life, and to reduce it solely to a scientific level diminishes that pleasure. Nevertheless, be sensible and modest. Train children to use a mere scraping of butter or margarine on bread or crackers, and encourage them to discard the fat on meat (give it to the birds).

Cholesterol

Cholesterol is a substance manufactured by the body, and it is found in many animal tissues. High levels in the blood – formed by eating too much saturated fat – have been associated with an increased risk of heart disease as a result of fatty deposits in the walls of arteries, known as atheroma. Some children as young as eleven years already show deposits from a high consumption of cholesterol. By thirty to forty years old they may run severe risk of early coronaries. The predisposition to deposit atheroma in the arteries is partly inherited, partly due to smoking, and much more common as yet in men. It is the major present-day cause of premature death. Those who can presume to have inherited a predisposition (all whose parents or grandparents suffered heart trouble) should give extra care to their diet throughout life, avoid smoking and take lots of exercise.

High level of cholesterol
1. Heart, liver, kidney, tongue, tripe, sweetbreads, brains. Serve small quantities (2–4 oz or 60–115 g) of liver or kidney once or twice a week for their otherwise invaluable contribution to the diet.
2. Fatty mince or meat, sausages, salami, ham, bacon, luncheon meat and tinned or prepared meats and pâté. Choose lean meats and cut off most of the visible fat. Drain cooked meat on kitchen paper after cooking.
3. Butter, creams, lard, dripping, cooking fat, suet, coconut and palm oils, cocoa, chocolate, cream cheese. Stilton and Cheddar type cheese. Serve cheese as an alternative to meat in a meal – as cheese salad, macaroni cheese etc – *not* in addition to meat at the end of a meal with butter and biscuits (an unhealthy habit).
4. Shrimps and prawns, fish roe.
5. Egg yolks. Serve three to five a week to small children, five to seven to teenagers, vegetarians, and expectant or nursing mothers; three to five for adults, but only one to three a week for those especially at risk – smokers, and those with a family history of coronary disease.

Fat Content of Common Food (as percentage of total)	
Food	**Percentage**
Oils	100
Lard, dripping	100
Butter, margarine	81
Nuts, double cream	50–60
Low-fat spread (margarine), bacon	40
Cheddar cheese, crisps, chocolate	35
Sausage, plain cake, chocolate biscuits	25
Lamb, pork, minced beef	20–30
Herring, mackerel, sweet biscuits, single cream	18
Avocado, soya beans	17
Ice cream, pastry desserts, chips, roast potatoes	11–14
Lean beef, veal, liver	10
Eggs, oats, salmon	8
Chicken	7
Milk, cottage cheese	4
Bread	1½–3
Pasta, rice	1
White fish, baked beans	½
Boiled or jacket potatoes, other vegetables and fruits	0

Although nuts, cheese and bacon are high in fat, their main other constituent is protein and they remain a useful part of the diet, unlike crisps, and excess oil, lard, butter etc.

Medium level of cholesterol
1. White, oily fish and smoked fish (not battered and fried).
2. Milk – avoid gold top. Allow 1–1½ pints (575–850 ml) per day for infants, children, teenagers, vegetarians and nursing mothers, ½ pint (300 ml) daily for others. Further quantities of milk are best taken as skimmed milk or low-fat yogurt for children, teenagers and adults.
3. Lean meats (best are poultry and rabbit).
4. Most margarine, cottage cheese, low-fat and curd cheeses, Edam and Gouda.
5. Peanuts, peanut butter, olives and avocados. Avoid peanut (groundnut) and vegetable oils in favour of low cholesterol oils (polyunsaturated).

Low level of cholesterol
1. Safflower, sunflower, corn and soya oils (use non-stick frying pan, so less oil is needed).
2. Polyunsaturated margarines (these are only 50 per cent poly, so even these should be taken in moderation. Train family to spread sparingly.)

Carbohydrates

These include sugars and starches and, technically, dietary fibre as well (the latter, which in the human gut cannot be broken down to provide energy or calories, is discussed later). Starches and sugars are a useful and often cheap source of energy. Those foods that contain carbohydrate as well as other useful nutrients in worthwhile quantities are those most recommended as part of the diet. Therefore bread (preferably brown), many cereals and potatoes, plus milk, fruit and other vegetables are considered infinitely preferable to sugar and refined cereals that provide little more than calories.

Sugars

Of all the items we eat sugar is alone in providing calories without providing some true nourishment such as protein, vitamins and minerals. In Britain we are now consuming 100 lb (450 kg) per head per year which is an average of 5 oz (150 g) for every man, woman and *child* daily. Most of this sugar is disguised: sweets, sugar-laden drinks, biscuits and cakes are more obvious, but much is contained in tinned and processed foods.

Both carob powder and maple sugar can be used as sweeteners, and they contribute vitamins and minerals, carob being particularly nutritious – a good source of calcium, phosphorus and fibre for those who crave sweet food. Nutritional recommendations are that we should aim at not more than 2–2½ oz (60–75 g) total daily intake of sugar for adults and less for small children.

Sucrose

Table sugar extracted from cane or sugar beet. It is present naturally in some fruits and other root vegetables – carrot, turnip, etc. It may be brown (less refined) or white, and there is only a marginal difference in food value, but the flavour of brown is much superior. The prime culprit in dental decay, table sugar provides calories, but contributes no other nutrient to the diet. It requires vitamins and minerals in its digestion, leeching out the body's reserves, yet providing none.

Lactose

The natural sugar in milk which provides all the energy a baby needs until about six months old. Sucrose sugar should never be added to a baby's feed as these additional calories are not needed.

Maltose

Sugar made when grain is fermented in beer-making. Malt, once popular with children, is not good for the teeth when given after meals, but its supplements of vitamins and minerals are useful for some on a poor diet, or with small appetite. Take *before* a meal.

Glucose

A simple sugar. Now preferred in place of sucrose sugar to sweeten infant baby juices, as it is less damaging to the teeth.

Fructose

A natural sugar, occurring in fruits, some vegetables and honey. It is the sweetest of the sugars, so less is required for a sweet effect.

Non-sugar sweeteners

Sorbitol is made from glucose, but is less quickly absorbed. It is used by diabetics, but is of no value to slimmers. Saccharin tastes sweet, but has no food or energy value. Five hundred times as sweet as sugar, it may be used by adults who have not learned to accept unsweetened fruits and drinks. Do *not* use for young children.

Starches

These are present in foods which are usually cooked. They include all grains, wheat, oats, rice etc. – in bread and breakfast cereals, for instance – and potatoes, pulses and some other vegetables. They are a cheap and healthy source of energy, so long as they are not heavily refined. Highly refined and modified starches contain little more than pure carbohydrate, and they are added heavily to many manufactured foods. These, like sugar, add very little to the diet, yet in their breaking down and use for energy a large quantity of B vitamins and minerals are needed.

Dietary fibre

Unlike some animals we are unable to digest the cellulose which forms the main structure of grains, vegetables and fruit – plus the skin, peel or husk. Although apparently useless, it is of immense value in its ability to absorb the other waste products of the body and speedily remove them. Some food with a good or high fibre content should be served at every meal.

Fibre Foods

Highest fibre content	Good fibre content	Low fibre content	No fibre
Bran cereal	Muesli	Chips, mashed or boiled	Butter
Baked and dried beans	Celery	potatoes	Cheese
Peas and sweetcorn	Most green vegetables	Tomatoes	Milk
Wholemeal bread	Apples and oranges	Lettuce	Fish
Wholewheat rye	Nuts	Cucumber	Eggs
crispbread	Most breakfast cereals	White bread	Meat
Prunes and dried fruit	Brown bread	White rice	Sugar
Bananas	Carrots		
Baked potatoes			
Green leafy vegetables			
Brown rice			

1. Fibre delays and to a small degree prevents the absorption of sugars in the blood. Useful for slimmers and those whose blood sugar level fluctuates quickly, giving changes of mood, and migraine.

2. It slows the absorption of sugars from the diet which will help protect the body from developing adult onset diabetes. Enables those who have diabetes to eat a more normal diet, since there is a steadier level of sugar in the blood, putting less demand on the body to produce insulin.

3. It protects the gut from the action of toxic waste products from the breakdown of foods, reducing the risk of all inflammations and complications of the gut – bowel cancer, appendicitis, colitis and stomach ulcers.

4. It keeps faeces soft, so they are readily expelled at least once a day. This causes less build-up of pressure in the lower bowel which will otherwise restrict the flow of blood from the legs and lower body back to the heart. This, in turn, would place stress on the walls of the veins, causing varicose veins and piles (haemorrhoids).

5. It reduces the absorption of cholesterol and is known to help protect against heart disease.

6. It is good for the teeth, as chewing encourages better flow of blood to the jaw, which is good for growing jaws, good for the gums, and reduces plaque on the teeth.

Minerals

There are fifteen minerals considered essential for the body, and at least a further five are believed to be necessary. Principal among them are calcium, phosphorus, magnesium, potassium and iron.

Calcium

Only part of the calcium we eat is absorbed. Adequate Vitamin D is needed for its absorption. About 99 per cent of the calcium in our bodies is in our bones and teeth; most of the remainder is essential for proper contraction of muscles.

Those most at risk from insufficient calcium are growing children of all ages and pregnant or lactating mothers. Expectant mothers whose diet is too low in calcium will first suffer some loss of calcium from their own bones (osteomalacia), which will be more pronounced with repeated pregnancies. They will suffer similarly when breast-feeding. It is less likely that the foetus will suffer as soon as the mother. Nevertheless, poor development of teeth, bones and skull can result if the mother's reserves are depleted.

Too early a move to mixed feeding can reduce a baby's intake of milk. This can put at risk the sound development of first and second teeth. It may reduce the skull size (and therefore brain) and result in stunted growth and rickets or bent leg bones. (Mothers should remember that all small children go through a period of the legs first appearing bow-legged, then knock-kneed before looking normally

Good Sources of Calcium, mg per 3½ oz (100 g)

Milk	120	Yogurt (natural)	180
Evaporated milk	290	Yogurt (fruit)	160
Dried skimmed		Sardines (canned)	550
milk	1,260	White fish	16
Cheddar cheese	860	White bread*	100
Cottage cheese	94	White flour*	138
Cream cheese	40	Wholemeal bread	28
* Extra calcium is added.			

straight at around seven years.) Cramp in the feet can be an indication of lack of calcium in growing children.

The children most likely to consume insufficient calcium are those who do not take milk, cheese or yogurt. For these, the recommended quantity of Vitamin D taken daily as a supplement will ensure maximum absorption from other foods. Adding plenty of dried milk powder to mashed potato, soups, puddings (crumble toppings for instance), and making home-made ice cream and mousses with evaporated milk, can discreetly and substantially increase the intake for the reluctant milk drinker.

The absorption of calcium is slightly inhibited by phytic acid and oxalic acid in some foods otherwise useful in the diet. Rhubarb, chocolate, coffee, tea and spinach are best avoided for the very young, and should be limited in growing children and expectant mothers. The early spring pickings of beet spinach are the highest in oxalic acid.

Phosphorus

Used in formation of teeth and bones and the release of energy. It is plentifully supplied in the diet. Too high a proportion of phosphorus to calcium, which occurs in cow's milk, but not human milk, can cause muscular spasms (tetany) in the first days of a baby's life. Cow's milk is therefore always modified for young babies.

Sources
Widely available in meat, fish, milk, eggs, nuts, grains and cereal foods, fruit and vegetables.

Magnesium

Present in bones and needed for conversion of calories into energy. It is part of chlorophyll, the green pigment in plants and vegetables. In pregnancy, there appears to be a greater need, so the diet should be plentiful in vegetables.

Sodium

Salt (sodium chloride) is needed for the balance of body fluids, and muscle and nerve activity. Surplus is passed out of the body in sweat and urine. Too high an intake is a problem in infants, especially under eight months, because they do not efficiently dispose of surplus through the immature kidneys. Salt should never be added to their food, and salty foods (ham, bacon, stock cubes, Marmite, gravy mixes) should be served only occasionally and salt itself only gradually in food after eight months.

Regular high salt intake is believed to contribute to high blood pressure. Those with a family history of this problem, strokes or water retention (oedema), should keep their salt intake at a low level throughout life. A little salt should be added to vegetables and other foods at the beginning of cooking, so it has plenty of time to dissolve for maximum good flavour, but it should never be sprinkled into or onto foods, when much larger quantities will be eaten. Do not put salt on the table or you will encourage this bad habit, but do add a very little to food to improve flavour.

Many modern children are being brought up on a diet of salted crisps, peanuts, sausages, canned and

---

Major Minerals

These are required in relatively large amounts, and have particular relevance to mothers and children.

	Calcium mg	Phosphorus mg	Potassium mg	Magnesium mg	Iron mg
Under 1 year	600	150	500	40	6
1–2 years	500–600	400	1,000	100	7
3–4 years	500–600	500	1,250	125	8
6–7 years	500–600	700	1,500	150	8
7–8 years	500–600	900	1,750	175	10
9–11 years	700–1,000	1,000	2,000	200	15
Teenager	700–1,300	1,300	2,500	350–500	15
Mother	500–600	800	2,500	350	12–14
Expectant Mothers	1,200	1,300	3,000	450	15
Lactating Mothers	1,500	1,300	3,000	450	15
Fathers	500–600	1,000	3,000	400	12

Also required are sodium chloride and sulphur.

other manufactured products. If they take this habit into adult life, there could be a great increase in high blood pressure and premature strokes. We are all advised to cut our salt consumption considerably.

Many pregnant women have a tendency to suffer fluid retention and high blood pressure. Keep salt intake low by choosing unsmoked and unsalted foods: pork not ham, herrings not kippers, plain not salted roast peanuts, etc. Be sparing when seasoning food, so that the whole diet has only a moderate salt content. Cramp in the feet and legs may be caused by lack of salt in athletes but is more likely to be from a low magnesium or Vitamin B_6 level in pregnancy so take more bran, wheatgerm, raw peanuts, brewer's yeast tablets and an otherwise good diet.

Potassium

The more salt eaten, the greater the depletion of potassium. A deficiency is only likely after gastro-enteritis or diarrhoea. Very severe loss can cause heart failure, but those with such an illness should already be receiving medical attention. Plenty of barley water, banana and apricot purée, carrot and parsnip, and fruit juices should aid a speedy recovery, and a good varied diet should be returned to as soon as possible.

Lack of potassium may contribute to colic in infants. If breast-feeding improve your diet. A change of milk feed may help some bottle-fed babies under four months. Choose the highest potassium to lowest sodium ratio. Foods which contribute most to potassium but least to sodium are fresh or home-cooked fruit and vegetables. Use for those over four to six months (add no salt). Introduce to diet slowly.

Diabetics (and those with a family history) should ensure a high potassium intake, which is needed in the proper use of sugars. The best way to ensure this, apart from giving plenty of fruit and vegetables, pulses, wheatgerm and unrefined grains, is to keep salt intake as low as possible. Choose unsalted breakfast cereal (check packet) whenever possible, and avoid salted foods.

Iron

Iron is mainly required by the blood for the carrying of oxygen, and lack of it can be one cause of anaemia. Iron is not easily absorbed, but Vitamin C can help. When resources are heavily depleted, after operations, or in pregnancy, iron tablets are given. It is most easily absorbed from liver and kidney. Other sources are dried apricots, dark green vegetables, eggs, other meats and cereal products.

Infants have most of their iron supplies for the first six months deposited in their bodies during the end of pregnancy. Those born prematurely will not have these reserves and may need extra prescribed. Breast milk contains little iron, but what there is appears to be well absorbed. Milk formulae contain more, but are not so well absorbed, and giving Vitamin C supplements will help efficient absorption.

Trace elements

These are known to be present in the body and tend to be needed in close relation to other minerals or vitamins. Lack of some of these minerals have been noted in a variety of mental or digestive disorders – diabetes, for example – but whether this is a result of deficiency or some people having a high requirement of them, or whether the disorder depletes the body, is not firmly established. As our knowledge of nutrition increases, we may become aware of links between mental illnesses and too low, or too high a level of minerals in the body (lead and cadmium, for instance), and the subtle interaction between minerals and chemicals in our food.

Zinc

Needed for bones and enzymes. Those taking very high levels of processed food may develop low levels. A deficiency could result in stunted growth and premature birth, but is not likely on a good diet. White flecks on nails and acne can indicate too low an intake.

Manganese

Used in the work of the enzymes, it is needed in larger amounts by diabetics and those with epilepsy. It is possible that those with a family history of these diseases should ensure a plentiful supply for their children. Wheatgerm and whole grains, tea, nuts and most vegetables provide manganese, also Epsom Salts (manganese sulphate). Wheatgerm daily would be a wise precaution for those whose need for manganese is high, also for expectant mothers and small children who are not drinking tea, whose vegetable consumption is low, and who are eating heavily refined cereals (only white bread and Rice Krispies).

Iodine

Required for the normal functioning of the thyroid gland and is richly supplied in all sea food. Choose sea fish – mackerel, herring, plaice, cod etc. – in

Trace Elements

Minerals required in very small quantities, but nevertheless important to ensure good health.

	Zinc mg	Manganese mg	Iodine mg	Copper mg
Infant	4	1	.04	.5
Childhood	6–8	3–15	.1	1
Teenage	15	20	.15	2
Adult	15	20–25	.2	2
Expectant or lactating mother	25	25	.2	2

Also required are fluorine, chromine and cobalt (figures taken from British and American recommendations).

preference to trout, once or preferably two to three times a week in pregnancy. The level of iodine in water, cereals and vegetables will vary considerably, depending on the soil in the area from which they come.

Low levels of iodine in pregnancy and early childhood can affect the IQ of the child and severe deficiency can cause mental retardation.

Copper

Required by enzymes, and a lack may contribute to anaemia. Cow's milk is a poor source, so a mixed diet is necessary for a baby by six months. Liver and green vegetables are given by this age and then followed shortly by all pulses (beans), wheat bran, avocado, and later mushrooms and dried currants. In pregnancy a healthy diet will ensure a baby is born with sufficient reserves unless premature.

Fluorine

A well-known protector of the teeth. Too much can cause brown mottling on the teeth, which is unsightly. If your local water supply has fluorine added, daily supplements may not be necessary. Children who swallow rather than spit out fluorinated toothpaste will certainly not require an extra dose. Seek your dentist's advice on supplements and teeth care for your area.

Vitamins

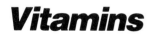

These substances are essential for good health and when too low in the diet can cause a number of minor ailments, a feeling of malaise, and infertility.

In children, growth and health are more obviously impaired.

The vitamins are separated into two groups. Vitamins A, D, E and K are soluble in fats or oils and may be stored to some extent in the body. The variety of substances that are in the B Vitamin group and Vitamin C are soluble in water. This group are more likely to be lost or leeched out in some cooking processes.

Vitamin A

Found in animal and fish livers (cod-liver oil), milk, cheese, butter and margarine in one form and, in a second form, beta-carotene, in green, yellow and orange vegetables and fruit. Carrots are a particularly good cheap source. The darker the colour of the vegetables – dark green and orange – the more Vitamin A they are likely to contain. Outer leaves of cabbages and sprouts etc. should not therefore be discarded, as they have greater food value. A little Vitamin A is present in chicken, peas, beans and oily fish.

Vitamin A is needed for the mucous membranes of the body, throat, nose, lungs, eyes, for the skin and tooth enamel. Severe deficiency can affect sight in dim light, but this is unlikely (it wasn't carrots which enabled pilots to see in the dark during World War Two, it was the invention of radar!). Lack of Vitamin A is likely in small fussy children who may be more prone to infections of the mucous membranes – colds, sore throats, bronchitis and infections of the skin and eyes. Beta-carotene is believed to protect the body from some forms of cancer, so serve carrots or dark green vegetables daily. In this form Vitamin A is not toxic.

Vitamin A is poisonous in too high a dose in cod-liver oil or Vitamin A supplements and these should only be taken at recommended levels.

Best Sources of Vitamin A, mcg per 3½ oz (100 g)	
Cod-liver oil	18,000
Cooked liver	17,200
Old carrots	2,000
Spinach, butter, margarine	900
Dried apricots	600
New carrots	500
Cheddar cheese	420
Dark green vegetables	350
Eggs	300
Apricots	250
Tomatoes, peaches	100

B Vitamin group

They are needed for growth and general good health. They are also needed for the enzyme system of digestion, which can affect appetite and digestive disorders. Most vegetables (except peas and beans), fruit, processed foods (except some breakfast cereal) and sugar are very low or contain no B Vitamins. (See faddy toddler's diet in Chapter Five.)

Vitamin B_1 (Thiamin)

Required for the gradual and continuous release of energy from carbohydrate foods. The more carbohydrate consumed, the more B_1 is required. Meat, milk, grains, pulses, eggs are good sources; brewer's yeast tablets are an excellent supplement.

Few lack B_1 but those at risk are alcoholics, plus small children eating large quantities of sweets, sugar, pop and refined processed foods. Those deficient in B_1 will have a poor appetite and general health, and lack a sense of well being.

Best Sources of Vitamin B_1 (Thiamin), mg per 3½ oz (100 g)		
Yeast extract	3	
Wheatgerm	1–2	
Fortified cereals	1.3	(approx.)
Raw peanuts	.9	
Pork	.58	
Oatmeal	.5	
Unpolished rice	.32	
Liver	.27	
Eggs	.27	
Peas	.25	
Roasted peanuts	.23	
Wholemeal bread	.23	

Vitamin B_2 (Riboflavin)

Needed for the use of energy in food, for the production of antibodies, and for the function and development of the brain. Plentiful in milk, meat and grains. Breakfast cereals are often fortified with B_2. It should be remembered that this vitamin is destroyed in sunlight, so that milk should not be left on the doorstep for long. Small faddy toddlers may be on a diet too low in riboflavin. Lack causes poor appetite, compounding their problem, and there may be sores round nose and corners of mouth. A plentiful supply is needed in pregnancy and is assured with a daily diet including 1 pint (575 ml) milk, an egg, plus meat, cheese and beans. It is linked to the proper absorption of iron.

Best Sources of Vitamin B_2 (Riboflavin), mg per 3½ oz (100 g)		
Liver	3.1	
Kidney	1.9	
Fortified cereal	1.4	(approx.)
Wheatgerm	1.3	
Cheese	.5	
Eggs, mushrooms	.47	
Most meat, dried beans	.2	
Milk	.15	
Some also present in nuts, brown bread and vegetables.		

Nicotinic Acid (Niacin in USA)

Its use by the body is similar to riboflavin. Lack causes poor health and vitality, sometimes sores and ulcers in the mouth, but is unlikely in those on a good normal diet. Small faddy toddlers on junk food, high fat and sugar diet could be at risk.

Best Sources of Nicotinic Acid, mg per 3½ oz (100 g)		
Yeast extract	67	
Liver, peanuts	20	
Kidney, sardines	10	
Fortified cereals	10	(approx.)
Beef, chicken, pâté	7–9	
Cheese, lentils	5–6	
Fish, pasta, mushrooms	4–5	
Egg	3–5	
Beans, peas	2–3.5	
Bread	2–2.5	
Milk	2	
Rice, potatoes	1.5	

Pantothenic Acid

Required for the liberation of energy; a deficiency causes fatigue, stomach cramps and the sensation of pins and needles. It may cause changes in the personality, like restlessness, irritability and fretfulness.

Refining and canning of food may cause one-third to three-quarters of the pantothenic acid content of food to be lost. Those on highly refined diets, high in sugar and fat, could be consuming too little. Fussy toddlers are especially at risk, and infants on tinned baby foods.

Pantothenic acid is needed by the adrenal glands. Insufficient can create poor functioning of these and lead to severe allergies being developed. During times of stress, excitement, and great activity, there is a greater need of this vitamin for the release of hormones. Stress plays an important factor in triggering allergic reactions, especially when insufficient pantothenic acid is consumed. For this reason, all who are predisposed to allergies – at least 25 per cent of the population – would be wise to consume plenty of pantothenic acid and ensure it in the diet of their infants and children. It is possible that some people require many times the level recommended for the average expectant mother or young child.

Best Sources of Pantothenic Acid, mg per 3½ oz (100 g)

Yeast extract, liver	8
Sweetbreads, heart, kidney, egg yolk	2
Mushrooms, peanuts, wheatgerm	2
Wholemeal bread	1.5
Cheese, meat, fish, beans, pulses, soya beans, cereals, bran	less than 1
Milk	.3

Royal jelly of bees contains 1.2 mg per teaspoon – the equivalent of ½–1 oz (15–30 g) liver, so liver is obviously a much cheaper source of this active ingredient against allergy.

Often those who are allergic appear to react to some of the very foods which are the best sources of pantothenic acid in the diet, and dropping these depletes their diet still further. Few are allergic to kidney and liver, however, which should be consumed very regularly if milk, cheese, nuts, beans, eggs or wheat are omitted because of allergy.

Vitamin B_6 (Pyridoxine)

This is required for use of protein in the diet and for haemoglobin in the blood. Needs are increased in pregnancy and for those taking the pill, where low intake could cause anaemia. This may also affect the foetal development. B_6 may also reduce nausea, dizziness, fatigue and headaches, cramp in the feet in pregnancy. When under extra stress, the need for B_6 is great, and insufficient is likely to cause such stress side affects as insomnia, irritability, depression, dandruff, sore mouth and skin rashes. Brewer's yeast tablets in addition to a good diet for one to two months before pregnancy should ensure greater fitness and less nausea in early pregnancy.

Lack of B_6 is believed to contribute to heart disease and diabetes.

Best Sources of Vitamin B_6 (Pyridoxine), mg per 3½ oz (100 g)

Brewer's yeast, wheatgerm	rich sources
Liver, kidney, mackerel	.8
Meat	.4–.8
Walnuts, wholemeal bread	.4
Fish	.2–.8
White bread	.08
Eggs	.05
Milk	.01

Sweetcorn, cabbage, sprouts and pulses are also good sources.

Vitamin B_{12} (Cyanocobalamine)

Required for bone marrow and other rapidly dividing cells, also for similar functions to B_1, B_2 and B_3. A deficiency causes pernicious anaemia and breakdown of nerve cells, through lack of meat, milk and eggs in the diet. B_{12} does not occur in plants. Vegetarians would be advised to take a supplement before and during pregnancy and childhood. It can affect fertility and brain development.

Best Sources of Vitamin B_{12} (Cyanocobalamine), mcg per 3½ oz (100 g)

Ox liver	111
Lamb's liver	84
Pig's liver	25
Eggs, white fish	1.7
Cheddar cheese, beef, lamb, pork	1.5
Milk	.3

Folic Acid

Works with B_{12} for division of cells, and deficiency may cause a form of anaemia. Folic acid is most important in pregnancy. A deficiency has been shown to be a major factor in spina-bifida and other malformations of the foetus. It is wise, therefore, to ensure a good diet before and during the first weeks of pregnancy, so that there is plenty of folic acid in the early stages of the developing embryo. This is the time when there is the greatest risk of abnormalities occurring in the division of cells, which results in congenital defects.

Mothers who have had several children in close proximity and those who have been on the pill will have particularly high needs of folic acid. One tablespoon of wheatgerm and two other good sources taken daily will amply supply needs.

Folic acid is destroyed in boiling, especially when Vitamin C is not present (much is dissolved in vegetable water and thrown away). Green vegetables need quick careful cooking with vegetable water used for sauces etc. Canned and other processed foods can be presumed to have little or no folic acid. Frozen vegetables, particularly peas, will still retain some.

Best Sources of Folic Acid, mg per 3½ oz (100 g)	
Wheatgerm, yeast extract	very rich source
Liver, kidney, dark green vegetables, raw peanuts, walnuts, raw cauliflower	1
Bread with added wheatgerm	.25–.75
Eggs, lettuce, mushrooms, tomatoes, oranges	.1–.2
Cheese, carrots, peas, bananas, grapefruit, potatoes	.01–.05
Meat, fish, white bread, apples, peaches, peas, milk	less than .01

Vitamin C

This vitamin is required for the absorption of iron, so particularly important in pregnancy, childbirth, at time of injury, burns and operations, to aid quick recovery and healing. Higher levels are needed by those who smoke or children whose parents smoke, children exposed to high levels of lead in the atmosphere of cities, and those taking aspirin regularly. Lack may cause anaemia and predisposition to infections. Cereals, instant, junk and processed foods, squash, pop, dairy products, meat (there are exceptions), fish, cheese and eggs contain no Vitamin C. Many small children are on a diet very low in this vitamin, and a daily supplement is necessary for such children to ensure their good health. Mothers with small children who are constantly picking up colds from schools would be wise to take high doses of Vitamin C as ascorbic acid powder if they are also caring for a small baby. The baby can be kept isolated from other germy members of the family for safety and Vitamin C might prevent the mother picking up the germ.

Vitamin C is very easily lost in cooking and in keeping food hot (in canteen food and school dinners, for instance). Unless fresh fruit is supplied these can generally be presumed to contain virtually no Vitamin C. Even in salads, the washing and handling of food usually means most of the vitamin is lost (except in tomatoes).

Great care should be taken preparing food. Never wash and leave green vegetables soaking in water. Shake dry after preparation and return to the fridge in a polythene bag. Do not slice or shred cabbage, cucumber, etc. in advance – most Vitamin C will be lost. Serve fruit raw, and avoid peeling fruit and vegetables whenever possible. Leave a potato (old *and* new) in its skin. It can then provide a useful cheap source of Vitamin C. Dark green leaves contain the most Vitamin C. Do not peel sprouts or discard outer leaves of other green vegetables unnecessarily. Dried vegetables contain no Vitamin C but if sprouted, their Vitamin C is returned.

Best Sources of Vitamin C (Ascorbic Acid), mg per 3½ oz (100 g)	
Blackcurrants	200
Brussels sprouts, broccoli, green pepper	85
Cauliflower, watercress	64
Raw cabbage, strawberries	58
Oranges	50
Canned orange juice, gooseberries	40
New potatoes, liver	30
Tomatoes, berries, pineapple, cooked cabbage	24
Tomato juice	17
Unpeeled apples, lettuce, bananas, bean sprouts	10
Old potatoes	8
Apples, peeled	5
Baked beans, peas, plums	3

Vitamin D

This vitamin occurs in very few foods – in fish, margarine, eggs, dairy foods and liver only – but fortunately in sunlight we manufacture much in exposed skin. This is of value in summer months and sufficient may be stored to help us through the autumn. For the rest of the year our diet needs to be relied on. Those with dark skins – West Indians or Asians – are not able to produce much Vitamin D in the poor northern sun, their skin being designed to protect them from prolonged and stronger sunlight. Dietary supplements are needed by them throughout the year, as well as by growing children in industrial cities and high-rise flats who receive little sunlight. All children up to five to seven years need Vitamin D supplements, especially in the winter months.

Vitamin D is required for the absorption and use of calcium for hardening bones and teeth. Babies, small children, and pregnant and lactating mothers are particularly at risk of lack, or their bones become very brittle, break with little pressure and teeth are lost. In infants, the skeleton and skull is poorly formed. Skull fracture becomes a real risk in toddlers and the child's weight when standing causes leg bones to bend and permanent deformity results. Both first and second teeth will be seriously damaged by a deficiency in the first five to seven years of life.

Vitamin D supplement is toxic if too much is taken. Measure Vitamin D drops for babies with great care. They should not be casually shaken out, but counted, and recommendations followed. Less may be given if your baby is exposed to sunlight in summer, but do *not* give extra in winter months just for good measure.

ONLY Sources of Vitamin D (Calciferol), mcg per 3½ oz (100 g)	
Cod-liver oil	212.5
Herring, kipper, eel, mackerel	22.2
Salmon, tuna (and other oily fish)	12.5
Margarine, low fat spread	8
Sardines	7.5
Evaporated milk	2.91
Eggs	1.5
Butter	1.25
Liver	.75
Cheddar cheese	.35
Milk	.05
Yogurt, cottage cheese	.02

Vitamin E

This is claimed to help fertility, reduce varicose veins, prevent scar tissue in burns, operations and when organs of the body and gut are damaged. It may be helpful in preventing atherosclerosis (hardening of the arteries), high blood pressure and in some forms of muscular dystrophy and cancer.

Vitamin E is needed for strong muscles, and in childbirth a lack may contribute to miscarriage or premature birth.

Vitamin E is normally widely available in our food. Slow growing plants contain more than the fast growing ones. Repeatedly heating cooking oils destroys Vitamin E. It has been found, surprisingly, that our need for Vitamin E is in fact *raised* when we take the polyunsaturated margarines recommended to reduce heart disease; and this is reflected in the new American recommendations.

At times of operations, childbirth, and for those

Vitamin E Recommendations (mg)	British	American
Under one year		5
1–2		8
3–4		10
5–6		12
7–8		13
9–11		14
Teenage		20
Mother	·3–5	25
Pregnancy	3–5	30
Lactation	3–5	30
Father	3–5	30

Best Sources of Vitamin E (Tocopherylacetate), mg per 3½ oz (100 g)	
Wheatgerm, vegetable oils	10–50
Olive oil, peanuts	5–10
Eggs, butter, cheese, ox liver, wholemeal flour, bread, oats	1–2
Whole-wheat breakfast cereals	0.5–1
Apples, carrots, peas, cabbage, white flour, bread, other cereals, meat, fish, milk, most fruit and vegetables	less than 0.15

predisposed to high blood pressure, heart disease, kidney and digestive disorders, it would be wise to take a high level. This may be best taken as a supplement of Vitamin E (D-alpha-tocopherol) after meals, where some fat or oil has been eaten to aid absorption. Premature babies may have poor stores of Vitamin E, a good reason for supplying them with breast milk and not formula, as this is a much better source. Vitamin E slightly reduces the need for oxygen. This is valuable at the time of birth when lack of oxygen can cause brain damage and blindness in babies if there is a difficult birth. Take a diet rich in Vitamin E before your labour.

Vitamin K

This is normally made by our intestinal bacteria and is needed for the clotting of blood – essential in childbirth and at times of accidents. We can make about half our needs.

The bacteria making Vitamin K are killed when you take oral antibiotics but can be best encouraged to develop again by taking a little yogurt at each meal. New babies are likely to be low in Vitamin K,

Vitamin recommendations

(Measurements in charts throughout the book are in micrograms (mcg), milligrams (mg) and grams (g).

	A mcg	B₁ mg	B₂ mg	Nicotinic Acid mg	B₆ mg	B₁₂ mcg	Folic Acid mg	Pantothenic Acid mg	*C mg	**D mcg	E mcg
Under 1 year	450	.3	.4	5	.4	2	.1	2	15	10	5
1–2	300	.5	.7	8	.7	3	.2	3	20	10	8
3–4	300	.6	.8	9	1.0	3	.2	4	20	10	10
5–6	300	.7	.9	10	1.3	3	.3	4	20	2.5	12
7–8	400	8	1.0	11	1.6	4	.3	5	20	2.5	13
9–11	575	1.0	1.2	14	2.0	4	.4	6	26	2.5	14
Teenage	750	1.4	1.7	18	5	6	.6	8	30	2.5	20
Mother	750	1.0	1.3	15	3	6	.5	10	30	2.5	25
Pregnant mother	750	1.0	1.6	18	4	8	.8	10	60	10	30
Lactating mother	1,200	1.1	1.8	21	4	8	.8	10	60	10	30
Father	750	1.2	1.7	18	4	6	.5	10	30	2.5	30

* American figures are double or treble these British recommendations.

** Requirements in winter months and for Asians and Africans is greater because less manufactured in the skin.

especially if premature or mother's diet was poor. They do not make their own in the first days of life and milk is a poor source. For your own safety and that of your child's, eat plenty of foods rich in Vitamin K during the weeks before childbirth, so that both of you are well supplied.

Best Sources of Vitamin K, mg per 3½ oz (100 g)

Cabbage, sprouts, cauliflower, spinach	up to 4
Beans, peas, carrots, potatoes, liver	up to 0.4

Normal daily requirement of Vitamin K is one helping of leafy vegetables or cauliflower daily during most of pregnancy, especially the last four weeks.

Fluid

This is required for the proper functioning of the kidneys which clear the body of waste. Lack of fluid may cause constipation and kidney damage.

Small babies are at risk of dehydration if the water content of the milk they drink is too low when bottles are made up with too much milk powder. Additional fluid is often only needed in hot weather and during and after vomiting and diarrhoea. Children need about 2 pints (1.1 litre) liquid per day. They usually take all they need, but they might need encouragement if they are ill or have colds when a high fluid intake is wise.

In pregnancy, there is a greater risk of cystitis, so an adequate fluid intake, about 3 pints (1.7 litres) daily, will keep this to a minimum. Those prone to cystitis, constipation, headaches, migraine and kidney infections should *always* aim at this intake, or even more. Drinking vast quantities when breast-feeding will not on its own assure a good supply of milk. Nevertheless, sitting down with a mug of milk, tea, coffee, etc. half an hour before feeding is helpful.

Tea and coffee

These are not recommended for young children for three main reasons (and, indeed, are not particularly good for adults in quantity).

1. They reduce the desire of children to drink milk or fruit and vegetable juices which are of considerable nutritional value.

2. They contain a kidney irritant (oxalic acid) found also in cocoa (chocolate), spinach, beet greens and rhubarb. The acid is less damaging when combined with calcium and magnesium but these make sharp crystals and can lead to kidney stones which will prevent the proper absorption of these minerals.

3. They both contain caffeine – a strong stimulant. Coffee has been found to contain further stimulants so that even decaffeinated varieties cannot be recommended for young children.

4. Drinking tea with a meal prevents the absorption of any iron consumed at the same time. Tea should be drunk well before or between meals for preference.

Water

Those living in hard-water areas have a lower risk of coronary heart disease. Whether this is due to components in soft water which increase risk, or whether the chalks in hard water – calcium and magnesium – prevent heavy metals like lead, mercury or cadmium being corroded into or dissolved in the water, is not proven. All drinking water should by-pass water softeners; if these are installed undesirable sodium is added.

Why a good diet is important

A good diet is vital from the earliest stage possible because deficiencies can cause the growing child to develop to less than his potential. Throughout life, many illnesses are at least partly self-inflicted through ignorance of the proper elements of diet. Increasingly, many of the foods we eat can be major killers, yet unlike tobacco they carry no Government health warning to advise us to severely limit their consumption.

The following diseases, of both childhood and adulthood, may all be related to the diet we choose.

Anaemia A diet deficient in iron, protein, Vitamin C, folic acid, Vitamins B_6 and B_{12}. It may also result from milk allergy.

Acne Lack of zinc, Vitamins A or E.

Appendicitis Lack of fibre in the diet.

Asthma, Eczema and Other Allergies Poor choice of food under seven months; bottle- not breast-fed.

Boils Poor diet with insufficient Vitamins B and C.

Cancer Lack of fibre and Vitamin A contribute to some cancers.

Colitis Lack of fibre in diet and bottle- not breast-fed in infancy.

Constipation Lack of fibre and fluid. Bad eating habits.

Cystic Fibrosis Inherited disorder, but a diet rich in iron, folic acid and Vitamin E can reduce risk.

Dental Troubles Poor dietary habits and lack of calcium and fluoride. Vitamins A, B, C and D affect quality of teeth and gums.

Diabetes Diet of expectant mother too high in nitrates and too low in Vitamin B_6 and magnesium can increase risk in childhood. Overweight and bad eating habits major cause in late onset. See Chapter Eight.

Diverticular Diseases Risk increased with low fibre and high sugar and fat intake.

Gastroenteritis More common in those bottle-fed.

Heart Disease Even before eleven years a bad diet too low in fibre and too high in saturated fatty acids, salt and sugar may cause cholesterol deposits in the arteries. High salt intake may affect blood pressure.

Kidney Diseases High salt intake, especially in the early weeks of life, and diet high in oxalic acid can create problems.

Health recommendations are that we should:

- Cut our average animal fat intake by 50 per cent
- Cut our overall fat intake by 25 per cent
- Cut our sugar consumption by 50 per cent
- Cut our salt consumption by 50 per cent
- Increase considerably our fibre intake

Chapter Two
Planning your pregnancy

It is ironic that even books on rearing hampsters advise a special diet before breeding to ensure normal and healthy young, yet future human parents, although they plan their families by means of birth control, give no thought to improving their diet, cutting out alcohol and smoking for a period *before* conception. *Both* parents should follow this advice so that neither sperm nor ova are damaged before conception and so that the embryo has the best chance for normal development. It goes without saying that the healthier the parents throughout their lives, the healthier the baby.

The health of a mother before conception can be crucial to her future child's health and her own well-being. During the period of conception, when the ovum and sperm fuse, and the first weeks of the developing embryo, the future child is very susceptible to damage. Any drugs, nicotine or alcohol can pass easily to the baby until the placenta is properly formed (by three months this will act as a filter to a large extent).

Before conception

Check that you have been immunised against German measles before you start a family to avoid the tragedy of contracting it in pregnancy and risking your child being born with a hearing, or other, defect.

If you are on the pill you should change to a different method of contraception three months before you wish to be pregnant to reduce risk of miscarriage or defects. Pill-users require more Vitamins B_2, B_6, folic acid, Vitamins C and E.

No drugs should be taken in pregnancy, especially during the early weeks. See your doctor three months before you hope to become pregnant if you take any pills, medicines or injections, or if you or any member of the family use eczema creams, so that only suitable types and doses can be prescribed.

Give up smoking before you are pregnant so that your baby will not suffer from carbon-monoxide and nicotine poisoning. They can permanently damage his brain and general health. Alcohol is now not recommended at any time during pregnancy, but a little occasionally is safer than a binge in the early weeks especially.

If you have problems conceiving, although there are many possible and probable reasons, it may be due to a lack of Vitamins A, B and E, which can all affect fertility. If you are overweight, have been anorexic, or if you are on a restricted diet, your fertility can be affected. Check with your doctor before you plan a family if you have a diet or weight problem. They could also affect a baby's development.

Foresight is an organisation to help parents ensure the optimum chance of having a healthy pregnancy and a healthy baby. It provides useful literature and is planning to open clinics. Hair analysis for determining metal and mineral levels in the body can be arranged – important for fathers as well as for mothers. Foresight strongly urge mothers to come off the pill for five to six months before pregnancy and use some other form of contraceptive while improving their health and reserves with a natural wholefood diet.

Foresight also recommend preconceptual supplements, and all details can be obtained from their Surrey base (see Appendix II). They market three different supplements which contain a very wide range of vitamins and minerals, and they recommend that they should be taken by *both* parents before conception, and continued by the mother during pregnancy and lactation. Do, however, discuss with your doctor before taking them after conception. These supplements are constantly monitored for maximum safety for your baby's future good health. These are available at health-food stores, some chemists, and in special cases even on prescription.

If this is your first child or there is about eighteen to twenty-four months' gap or more between each child – even if you have breast-fed for up to one year of this – there is plenty of time to build up reserves on a good normal diet. If, on the other hand, you have two children in under one year to fifteen months, or have a number of children with a relatively short gap between each, it is of great importance that you have a diet of very high nutritional value to maintain your own health, and are able to produce a really healthy child with a reduced risk of nausea and miscarriage (a good diet before pregnancy rich in B vitamins is the best prevention of nausea, so plan ahead). Lack of these reserves could be one of several reasons why younger children in a family are normally less intelligent than the first one.

Planning pregnancy is always wise. A mother may have taken a wide range of unsuitable items before she realises she has missed her first period. It is during the first six to eight weeks that all the organs of the body, limbs and face begin their separate development. Damage at this very sensitive stage through drugs, illness or poor diet or a combination of these are thought to contribute to a very wide range of malformation of limbs, cleft palate, defects of heart, lungs, eyes, ears and, of course, the brain.

After conception

Your own long-term health and that of your child can be affected by your diet at this time. There is no reason why you should lose your teeth and figure and end up with stretch marks and varicose veins, aged and fatigued. The prevention of all of these rests almost entirely in your own hands.

Your baby's teeth and bone structure, general good mental and physical health, freedom from allergies and intellectual potential are not only dependent on hereditable factors, but can be modified by an ideal maternal diet. To help improve this, free or cheap supplements are available and should be taken from the earliest advised opportunity. The early months of a baby's development in the womb are those most critical: exposure to some chemicals, smoking, maternal illness, drug taking, can all cause risks which are increased if the diet is poor, so ensure the best possible diet during the early stages and throughout.

A healthy diet at conception

1. Drink two mugs of weak tea or hot water first thing in the morning.
2. Drink a minimum of 3 pints (1.7 litres) liquid a day, more if needed.
3. Take 1–2 tablespoons bran and wheatgerm with breakfast cereals.
4. Eat liver once a week at least.
5. Eat only five eggs per week maximum. You may wish to avoid egg white which is constipating if you have a serious problem.
6. Eat fish two to three times a week.
7. Eat leafy green vegetables every day, beans and lentils regularly.
8. For snacks, eat dried figs, apricots, raisins (preferably sun-dried) etc., not sweets or cakes.
9. Choose wholemeal or whole-grain cereals, crackers, rice, bread, pasta.
10. Keep fat intake low, with not too much cheese unless low fat or cottage.
11. Boil or bake scrubbed potatoes in skins. Avoid roast potatoes and chips.
12. Eat skins of washed fruit and vegetables when possible.
13. Serve fruit and vegetables raw as often as possible.
14. Eat a little bran or bran cereal before going to bed.
15. Take more exercise – some yoga exercises are particularly helpful.

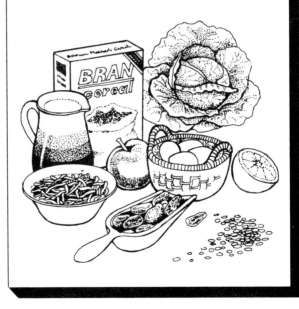

A healthy diet during pregnancy

If you develop a classic passion for something unusual – but good – like apricots, strawberries or watercress, indulge yourself happily, but if it is a passion for chocolate or sticky buns, do not. You need at this time to eat sensible food more frequently to keep your blood sugar level up, so plan at least six good small meals a day.

On waking: Before getting out of bed, have a cup of milk, or tea, and a wholemeal cracker, digestive biscuit or honey sandwich made with wholemeal bread.

Breakfast: Whole-grain cereal, muesli or porridge, plus wheatgerm and fruit juice.

Elevenses: Milk and a wholemeal sandwich filled with egg, meat, peanut butter, sesame seed spread, liver pâté or cottage cheese, or a fruit and nut snack of raw peanuts, walnuts, dried apricots and raisins (easy to take to work).

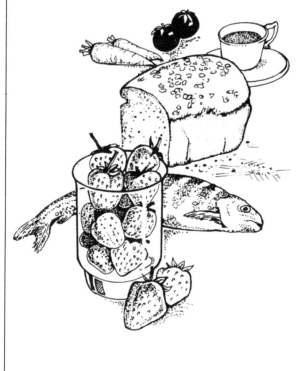

Lunch: *Choose from the following.*

Meat — Choose liver once a week. Vary meats, include pork and poultry, kidney, lean beef and lamb, a little bacon or ham, and avoid processed meats as far as possible.

Fish — Choose oily fish – mackerel, herring, sardine – with kippers and smoked fish occasionally. Eat plenty of white fish, grilled, poached or baked (not fried).

Cheese — Plenty of cottage cheese, with some Cheddar or curd cheese, especially if meat and fish are limited. Avoid cheese spread and processed cheese.

Pulses — Plenty of lentils, split peas, all beans, including canned beans. Good in soups, casseroles etc.

Vegetables — Aim at one green vegetable daily: cabbage, spinach, sprouts, watercress etc. Potatoes cooked in their skins. Avoid chips and limit roast potato. Include carrots regularly, cooked or raw. Plan one salad a day.

Egg — One per day.

Tea: Tea, plain yogurt or milk, and one or two of the following: fresh or frozen fruits, nuts, wholemeal sandwich of peanut butter, curd cheese, sesame seed spread, tomato or watercress. Wholemeal fruit loaf or scones.

Dinner: As lunch, one course.

Bedtime: Milk drink – Horlicks, Ovaltine, or Bournvita, not coffee or cocoa. Apple crumble, baked custard, fairly low calorie dessert (perhaps left over from the family's lunch or dinner).

Nutritional Daily Requirements for Pregnant Mother

Calories	2,400	Nicotinic acid	18 mg
Protein	60 g	Pantothenic	
Calcium	1,200 mg	acid	10 mg
Iron	15 mg	Vitamin B_6	3 mg
Magnesium	450 mg	Vitamin B_{12}	8 mcg
Zinc	25 mg	Folic acid	0.8 mg
Vitamin A	750 mcg	Vitamin C	60 mg
Vitamin B_1	1 mg	Vitamin D	10 mcg
Vitamin B_2	1.6 mg	Vitamin E	5–30 mg

Recommended Supplements and Treatments

As a result of recent tests few artificial supplements are now recommended in pregnancy. Mothers are advised to rely on a good diet before conception and during pregnancy as the safest protection for themselves and child. Only take vitamin and mineral supplements in pregnancy after consulting your doctor.

1. Tablets may be supplied which contain Vitamins A, C, D, plus calcium and iodine. They should be taken at a meal-time once a day.

2. Supplements of folic acid and iron are sometimes prescribed (overdoses of these are highly dangerous to toddlers so store with care). Eat food high in folic acid in early pregnancy.

3. Milk is supplied by voucher for 1 pint (575 ml) a day only for those with two children under five or with special circumstances (see Social Security office).

4. All prescriptions are free.

5. All dental treatment is free.

6. Fluoride. There are varied views on the taking of fluoride during pregnancy. It does improve the baby's future teeth. Consult doctor on latest views on safety for your baby's general health.

Vitamins A, B, C and E can be particularly valuable during pregnancy, so any extra intake is wise. For Vitamin A eat carrots or dark green vegetables daily. For Vitamin B take brewer's yeast tablets with added B vitamins (do not take as active dried yeast for bread-making) or wheatgerm daily. For Vitamin E, take D-alpha-tocopherol capsules after meals (but not at meals when iron tablets are taken). Extra doses of Vitamin C (ascorbic acid powder) at any time you are exposed to infections may help to protect from cold, flu etc. Buy from a chemist or reputable health-food shop, and check with your doctor or midwife if you are unsure what you may safely take.

Weight gain

This is essential in pregnancy to ensure good development of the child. The weight is made up of some fat deposits to be used in breast-feeding (and which will be quickly lost later on a careful diet), the weight of the foetus, placenta and amniotic fluid (lost at the time of birth), the weight of enlarged uterus (lost shortly after the birth, as it naturally shrinks), and the breasts. Your weight will be monitored and you will be advised if it is too great at any stage at the ante-natal clinic. The correct weight gain will suggest to the doctor that progress is satisfactory, but he will find it difficult to judge if the increase is from empty calories – from sweets and cakes – or from the proper deposits of essential nutrients for future good health of mother and child. There should be negligible gain in weight the first three months; between fourteen and thirty weeks is the time of major weight gain. The total needed in pregnancy is around 18 lb (8 kg), so an ideal aim for the average sized mother would be between this and 20–24 lb (9–12 kg) increase. Much more than this would be excess fat or fluid retention, and thus undesirable.

If you are going to have twins (or more!), the same well chosen diet, rich in proteins, vitamins and minerals, should ensure they are born near full term. They will otherwise lack the reserves of iron and other minerals to help good development. Be doubly – or trebly! – meticulous about your diet. Your doctor or clinic will advise on suitable weight gain.

For an easy delivery

A good diet rich in protein, potassium and Vitamin E should ensure strong healthy muscles for a speedy and easy delivery. It will help keep tissues elastic and reduce risk of episiotomy or tearing at birth. Vitamins C and K, calcium and iron will help ensure good clotting of the blood after birth with minimum bleeding or subsequent anaemia. Calcium and Vitamin C are believed to reduce pain.

Your baby will also need a constant supply of energy at this time to last through birth and until he is fed, so you should have plenty of milk to drink; yogurt, bread, cheese and fruit make good snacks in early labour. Make some cheese sandwiches to take with you to hospital in case you (or your husband) feel hungry later, if the first stage of labour is prolonged. Eating too near delivery is likely to make you sick as the body is not able to digest food well in the second stage of labour.

(And those cheese sandwiches may come in useful later: one of the commonest memories *after* childbirth is of extreme hunger!)

Foetal health

The belief that only a mother's health suffers by poor diet in pregnancy is not correct. She may appear relatively healthy while her foetus is malnourished or damaged through lack of care.

Alcohol

Large amounts of alcohol will definitely be dangerous to your developing baby. It is now believed that even one glass of wine could increase the risk of damage to a baby, especially if the mother is not on an ideal diet or in good health. Advice has previously therefore varied from the very cautious, saying no alcohol, to drinking small quantities of wine or beer with a meal, from those who feel the risk is minimal and that the advantages of the mother being more relaxed outweigh the disadvantages. American research is quite conclusively in favour of no alcohol, most particularly in the first eight to twelve weeks of the embryo's development, when risks of deformity, miscarriage, or stillbirth are much increased. Later drinking of alcohol in pregnancy is believed to affect the development of the foetal brain. It is quite common for a mother to develop an aversion to alcohol while she is pregnant, in which case giving it up entirely will be less of a hardship than previously imagined. It is particularly unwise for older pregnant mothers (35+) to drink on a regular basis. Their babies are already at greater risk.

Drugs

Only those drugs prescribed for you with pregnancy in mind should be taken. If your pregnancy was not planned and you did not see your doctor before you were pregnant, see him promptly. Some people will have to take drugs in pregnancy for long-term conditions, diabetes and thyroid deficiency for instance. The type and dose used may need changing with your baby's health in mind.

Avoid patent remedies for colds, flu and other minor ailments. Only the recommended vitamin and mineral supplements should be taken in addition to a good diet to ensure the best possible health for your baby. Remind your doctor that you are pregnant when you attend his normal surgery for any ailments and he will then be sure to only prescribe suitable drugs for you in this condition.

Some creams and ointments for external use are not suitable for an expectant mother to use or administer. Avoid steroid/cortisone preparations on yourself or other members of the family until you have checked with the doctor.

Coffee, strong tea, cocoa, Coca-Cola and chocolate all contain the drug caffeine. Avoid it in pregnancy and try herbal teas instead, which will reduce nausea. Many mothers develop a natural aversion to coffee. Do not wait to see if you do, but give it up so that your baby is not exposed in the earliest weeks, and drink decaffeinated later, if you must.

X-rays

X-rays could damage the developing foetus, so advise and remind your doctor and dentist you are pregnant before treatment. It is essential both know before taking X-rays, giving anaesthetics or drugs, so that only suitable treatment is given.

Smoking

Many full-term babies born to mothers who smoked all through pregnancy appear as much as a month premature at birth. Their birth weight is well below average and any baby who is below his ideal weight at birth is going to have to have far greater care taken of him in the first months or even years of life. Smoking decreases the circumference of the skull (and therefore the size of the brain) at birth. This could decrease the intellectual potential or even cause brain-damage in severe cases.

Smoking increases the nutritional needs of the mother, and also often decreases appetite for essential food. Vitamin C is needed in much greater quantities. This will affect the iron absorbed by the mother for her baby's deposits, which have to last him the first six months of life, when his iron intake will be low.

Carbon-monoxide in the blood of a smoking mother will pass into her baby's bloodstream. This produces oxygen starvation which results in the poor development of the foetus.

Kitchen household and garden products

A mother's intake can be through her lungs and skin, not just her mouth. Lead from scraping down old paintwork, exhaust fumes or inadequate washing of hands, fruit and vegetables in industrial areas can affect the brain development of the foetus. Leave home-decorating to others if possible, or only work in a very well ventilated atmosphere. Spirit bases of paints and the colour pigments could create a risk.

Avoid inhaling all strong chemicals, and use of aerosols should be kept to a minimum. Be especially careful of all garden chemicals. Many advise the use of gloved hands and other precautions. Insufficient is known concerning many chemicals and their affect on the foetus, so it is wisest to prevent all contact. Those who cannot avoid some exposure should take particular care in the first twelve to fifteen weeks of pregnancy and should take plenty of Vitamin C and a good diet to minimise the effect on their body or foetus.

Permitted food additives and colourings

A wide range of chemicals are added to foods as colouring, flavouring, anti-oxidants, preservatives, stabilisers, emulsifiers, etc. to make manufacture easier, distribution less hurried, and to tempt and titillate the purchaser into buying products that are profit-making, but not necessarily nutritious. Those that are permitted, or considered comparatively safe in this country, may not be considered safe in another country; the red colouring, amaranth, is banned in the USA, for instance (often used in sweets).

We do not know enough about the combined effects of these substances (they are tested singly for safety standards). Try to choose a diet low in food additives, although it is not necessary or practical to avoid them altogether. Make the major part of your diet fresh or frozen foods that are not highly processed. For example, serve potatoes boiled or baked in their skins for ease rather than use instant mashed potato, or frozen chips. Serve wholemeal bread (avoid part-cooked packet bread). Make your own soups, sauces, cakes, etc. (avoid packet mixes). Wash all fresh vegetables well to remove traces of crop spraying etc.

Problems in pregnancy

Many of the conditions and problems associated with pregnancy can be avoided completely or at least alleviated, by eating properly (see previous pages for good diets).

Nausea

Doctors will be reluctant to give medication for this, especially in the first three months, unless the condition is very severe. In this case prolonged sickness would of course mean that the mother and foetus may become lacking in essential nutrients.

Good nutrition before pregnancy will provide the best protection from nausea, especially a diet including plenty of wheatgerm, liver, whole grains, pulses, fish and citrus fruits. From the earliest days of pregnancy and at the first signs of the slightest nausea, plan your food intake very carefully.

Avoid coffee – you will probably not like the taste anyway – and have very weak tea, or herbal teas instead. Many of these will aid digestion and reduce nausea. Try peppermint and lime flower. Avoid sweets, sweet foods (except honey), cakes, sweet puddings. You may crave these and they may briefly appear to stem nausea for perhaps half an hour, but greater nausea may follow or general nausea increase. It is better to nibble a little wholemeal toast or whole-grain cracker.

Plan your diet with many small meals – about six, including good snacks (see page 30). Make sure your whole-food intake is highly nutritious. Plan some protein at each meal, but possibly only one course – even at main meals. Puddings, if not too sweet, can be set on one side until the next 'snack' time. Some may find it better not to drink and eat at the same time. Try drinking half an hour after a meal, but remember to drink enough during the day – six large cups a day or more.

It is important that the first food of the day should be taken in bed. If your husband cannot bring this up for you, then have a box of suitable biscuits, plus a tray and kettle by the bed, or a thermos. Weak, milky tea suits some, but herbal teas are a good alternative. Get up about half an hour or more after this.

Eat a little food with a milky drink just before you go to bed so that early-morning nausea is reduced.

If you actually vomit, lie or sit down afterwards and have a small quantity of food to nibble as soon as possible. Wholemeal toast (no butter at first) with honey, eaten very slowly, should help you to recover. Increase your intake of wheatgerm and take brewer's yeast tablets, both rich in B_6 and other B vitamins, which can help to counteract nausea.

Fried foods, hot spicy foods and chocolate may increase nausea. Sudden activity, shock and going from a warm room into a cold atmosphere are all likely to cause nausea. Be particularly wary of eating a large meal at a restaurant, or at a friend's, followed by a cold or difficult journey home in the first three months of pregnancy. It is important that otherwise the diet remains healthy but not too fattening. Some foods good in themselves can be taken in too great a quantity. Milk should be restricted to 1 pint (575 ml) fresh whole milk – any more should be taken as skimmed milk, because of the weight problem.

Severe sickness should always be discussed with a doctor, but many women can manage mild nausea adequately. Those with severe nausea may have to nibble food half-hourly throughout the day to prevent sickness. Choice of food needs great care, and any mother eating foods at more frequent intervals will be much more prone to dental decay. Teeth will need brushing more than twice a day to keep in good condition.

Indigestion, wind and heartburn

These are frequently a problem in pregnancy. A well-balanced diet before and during pregnancy should reduce this. Often the first foods that are given up to attempt to reduce this (beans, lentils, cabbage and whole-grain cereals) are those highest in the vitamins which would most help to return the digestion to normal. Eat small meals low in fat to reduce all three problems. Avoid well-cooked cabbage and sprouts. These are more, not less, indigestible than raw or lightly cooked vegetables.

Many herbs aid digestion. Use mint, parsley, dill, fennel, sage and savory liberally. They should be added fresh or dried to broad beans and all recipes using dried beans and lentils to reduce wind. Start each meal with 1–2 tablespoons of plain yogurt. Very slowly increase the wheatgerm taken daily, and gradually start taking brewer's yeast tablets. Do not add bicarbonate of soda to green vegetables or take anti-acid tablets. Take only medicaments prescribed specifically for pregnancy, apart from the natural supplements of wheatgerm and brewer's yeast tablets.

An increase in fibre in the diet and more exercise will also help. Remember to keep all meals very small, taking six or more snacks or meals with the total daily intake, providing a balanced diet.

Constipation in pregnancy

The extra pressure of the enlarging uterus makes constipation a greater problem and more likely for those who are prone. This additional pressure increases the likelihood of piles and varicose veins developing. The severe pressure on the veins carrying the flow of blood away from the legs and lower regions, results in blood vessels becoming enlarged below the womb and rectum.

Sufficient fluid, especially at the beginning of the day, and the addition of broad bran to the diet are the most affective solutions. Natural broad bran is the most efficient bran cereal at counteracting constipation, although perhaps not the most palatable. If a normal high fibre diet is insufficient alone, take 1 tablespoon of this bran daily. Add to other cereals, soups, fruit purées, casseroles, etc. Gradually increase the bran if this quantity is insufficient, but otherwise keep to the minimum level for good results.

Varicose veins and piles in pregnancy

Avoiding constipation as above is vital. Overweight will put a great strain on your circulatory system. Try to keep to your recommended weight gain, or not more than 24 lbs (12 kg).

Other golden rules are never ever to sit cross-legged. Never stand when you can sit working in the kitchen or ironing, for instance. Never sit when you can lie or, at least, sit with your legs up – watching television, reading etc. When standing, washing up or in other activities in the kitchen, slowly rock weight from one leg to the other. Wear support tights at the first sign of trouble. During pregnancy, maintain a diet high in Vitamins C and E. Take supplements of wheatgerm and Vitamin C (ascorbic acid) powder.

Stretch marks

Overweight and/or diet poor in Vitamin C can both contribute to an increase in stretch marks. Aim at an ideal weight gain and healthy diet.

Toxemia

Two main symptoms of this are high or fluctuating blood pressure, and albumin (protein) in the urine. These will be carefully monitored throughout pregnancy by your doctor. His findings are very much in your hands, and every mother can reduce the chance of toxemia and its side effects with sensible care. High blood pressure is much less likely in a diet low in salty foods (ham, kippers, table salt etc.) and high in potassium (fruit, vegetables, meat, whole-grain foods). Albumin in the urine is a serious problem, not only as a symptom of toxemia, but because protein consumed by the mother is needed by both herself and her baby. If these are lost in the urine, both may suffer from protein deficiency. The diet should be quite high in protein foods during pregnancy. In addition to ¾–1 pint (575 ml) of milk, 4 oz (115 g) meat or fish, eggs, cheese, peanut, wholemeal bread, whole-grain cereal or pulse vegetables should be taken daily, and liver at least once a week.

The protein foods also contain a substance called cholin, which helps protect the body against all aspects of toxemia and high blood pressure. It is needed in much greater quantities by those whose diet is high in refined sugar, alcohol and fats – a further reason why these should be kept low.

Anaemia

During the last few weeks of pregnancy your baby will draw from your body sufficient stores of iron to last him the first six months of his life when he will absorb little from his diet. To ensure you do not suffer anaemia while you are pregnant, nor after the birth (when you will lose more iron in blood), it is important that your diet is well supplied with not only iron (from liver, kidney, meat and leafy green vegetables), but also Vitamin C to aid its absorption and speed healing. Vitamin B_{12} and folic acid are also important in protecting against anaemia which will cause fatigue in pregnancy and greater risk of post-natal depression later, after the baby is born.

Working mums

Many pregnant mothers will have to rely on canteen and snack bars for their midday meal, where the choice of food can be very limited – largely pies, pasties, chips, stodge in general, synthetic soups and drinks. Many such eating places offer no fruit or fresh vegetables, and more nutritious alternatives can often be far too expensive. You may be able to opt for taking a packed lunch – a wholemeal roll and cheese plus fruit can be prepared in a moment the night before, or in the morning before you leave for work, and it makes an ideal lunch. If this is not practical, try at least to select from a menu a cheese or egg salad wholemeal sandwich or roll, cheese on toast or beans on toast. Avoid carbonated drinks and choose milk or real fruit drinks instead, with fresh fruit or yogurt, if they have it, for dessert.

If the choice is really limited for a balanced lunch, take well planned *snack* food for tea or coffee breaks: avoid cakes and biscuits, and provide your own fresh or dried fruit, tomato, sticks of raw carrot, celery or cucumber, cheese, yogurt or fruit drink to ensure a better diet.

Look at the suggestions for packed lunches for children in Chapter Six; many of them can be adapted for a good lunch for a mother-to-be.

Planning six small meals a day may sound like hard work to a busy mum. Basically, it just means choosing nutritious snacks like fruit for mid-morning and mid-afternoon break instead of eating junk foods, biscuits and sweets, plus leaving your evening meal pudding to eat at bedtime.

Chapter Three
Feeding your baby

Most mothers are well prepared for childbirth – a day's activity (hopefully) – but do not receive enough information on the care and feeding of their baby. Many new mothers have neither bottle-fed a baby nor even seen a baby breast-fed before their own arrives.

During the first five to six months of your baby's life milk will be almost the sole food he requires; you will have plenty of time to think about solid feeding later. You need as much information as you can get on breast- and bottle-feeding before you have your baby; you need time to prepare your nipples before birth, to improve your diet, and you need to know where to turn for good information and advice.

Apart from considering the advantages and disadvantages of breast- and bottle-feeding it is probably a good time now to review your family eating habits. These your child will start to acquire in his first year and it may be that the way you eat is not an ideal pattern for the next generation. Possibly both mother and father will need to change their eating pattern and choice of food to set an example to their children. Learning to drop bad habits takes time, so plan ahead.

When planning future feeding it is vital to remember that much can be done to prevent a very wide range of allergies by a careful choice of food in the early months (see Chapter Nine if allergies run in your family).

Vitamin supplements for babies

Government vitamin drops are recommended as a daily supplement for all babies from five weeks. A full dose is five drops which supplies Vitamins A, C and D. Additional supplements may also be given if a baby is premature or has special milks supplied by a doctor.

Breast-feeding

We are at last moving into an era when breast-feeding is once again fashionable. With their greater feeling of liberation and confidence, women can admit to the pride they have in their bodies and can allow themselves to enjoy the pleasurable physical sensation of breast-feeding, not feeling embarrassed to do it in front of others. The next generation will hopefully see breast-feeding as a normal part of life without any awareness of the prudery that dominated the past. Breast-feeding should be demonstrated in schools to all fifteen-year-olds in courses on biology, preparation for life and child care, for *both* boys and girls, so that the proper function of the breast is appreciated by all (a husband's views can be very influential).

Through lack of sufficient help and proper advice many mothers who start to breast-feed give up in two to four weeks. Although this short period will have been of immense value to a baby, it is sad that so many do not persevere, or do not seem to enjoy it. Alas, most of us cannot turn to our mothers or grandmothers for advice in the art of breast-feeding. Nor can we always reliably turn to all doctors, nurses, midwives, health visitors etc., as their training might have been completely lacking in the proper management of breast-feeding. Some have acquired only very basic knowledge, and many have never actually breast-fed themselves. Fortunately there is a gradual increase in the numbers who are expert in this field, and who can fill the gap in information, advice and personal support if your local medical care is lacking. One such organisation is La Lèche League which was founded to promote breast-feeding and to help mothers breast-feed successfully; they have a large network of counsellors throughout the country, and offer a twenty-four-

Advantages of breast-feeding

1. Breast-feeding increases the level of the hormone prolactin, which is often described as 'nature's tranquilliser', and which improves the maternal instinct and bonding between mother and child. A further hormone, oxytocin, also helps the womb to return to normal quickly, reducing blood loss. It is released when your baby sucks.

2. Breast-fed babies are a greater pleasure to the senses. Their skin is softer and smoother and freer of rashes. They smell nicer, and their breath, posseting (regurgitation) and nappies do not have an unpleasant odour.

3. Breast milk is perfectly formulated to meet a baby's requirements. It changes substantially from the colostrum of the first few days to the early breast milk and then to the more satisfying milk which develops at around three months to meet the baby's varying and increasing needs.

4. Breast-feeding is very convenient. No matter where you are or what hour of the day or night, you can pick up your baby to feed him. At night have your baby near you. You can then pick him up and tuck him in bed with you to feed him and both of you will quickly go back to sleep – no need to change him or even return him to his cot (so long as neither you nor your husband are on sleeping pills, drunk or very overweight, there is no risk of suffocating him).

5. Breast-feeding is cheaper than bottle-feeding, as no formula milks or sterilising solutions are needed. You will need to eat well and wisely even if you are not breast-feeding in order to maintain good health and prevent fatigue and depression.

6. Breast-feeding is safer than bottle-feeding, as no sterilisation is needed; the breasts are just washed normally each day and dried. Breast milk supplies antibodies and antitoxins to help protect the infant from infections and poisons. Babies will be much less prone to gastroenteritis and other illness. It is very unwise not to breast-feed for the first five days of a baby's life, even if you do not intend to continue any longer. The supply of protective agents is particularly high in your milk at this time.

7. Breast-feeding greatly reduces the risk of all allergic conditions – asthma, eczema etc. – particularly if the infant is given only breast milk until seven months and solid foods chosen very carefully from four to seven months. Even a few weeks' breast-feeding reduces risk of allergic problems.

8. Colostrum is very high in Vitamin A; infants have no store of this at birth and it is essential for the health of mucous linings of the lungs, nose and eyes. This intake creates less risk of chest infections and bronchitis.

9. Enzymes present in unheated milk – straight from the breast – assist with hardening of the bones and teeth. Heat and storage destroy other nutrients in milk.

10. More body weight of breast-fed infants is muscle and less fat deposits, and this reduces the tendency to overweight in later life.

11. Breast milk is high in unsaturated fatty acids, especially linoleic, essential for proper cell growth. Some cow's milk formulas are being improved to include fats of vegetable origin which contain more linoleic acid.

12. Sucking in breast-feeding is stronger than that on a conventional teat on a bottle. The new orthodontic teat is hoped to minimise this disadvantage in bottle feeding. Proper sucking at the breast promotes better development of jaw and facial bone structure, sinuses etc. Children should develop with less risk of overcrowded teeth, better articulated speech, and with more attractive tone of voice.

13. Protein molecules in breast milk are a quarter the size of doorstep cow's milk protein, and both protein and calcium as a result are better absorbed in breast milk. This gives optimum growth of the skull and development of the brain and therefore IQ potential.

14. The better absorption of calcium and certain other minerals – magnesium and zinc for instance – will help the baby to be less highly strung and nervy.

15. Breast-feeding does not drain your strength as formerly believed. Caring for a new baby is very tiring, and cleaning, sterilising and making up feeds is more likely to make you weary than sitting down and putting your feet up to breast-feed baby regularly.

16. You have one free hand when breast-feeding to play with your baby, to give a cuddle to another child or your husband, pick up a book or have some refreshments yourself.

17. Breast-feeding is considered to reduce the risk later in life of heart disease, allergies, bronchitis, colitis, multiple sclerosis, cancer and the development of addictions to smoking, drugs and alcohol.

hour service. The National Childbirth Trust also offers breast-feeding help through a promotion group, and there are local branches. (See Appendix II for addresses.)

A healthy diet for breast-feeding

Breast-feeding is no more tiring than bottle-feeding if a mother's diet is adequate. Caring for a baby does make extra demands, and no matter how she feeds her baby she is likely to feel very tired during the first few weeks after birth. A poor diet will result in a poorer quality of breast milk.

Foods to take

Vitamin B requirements are high at times of stress and when sleep is lost. Eat plenty of meat, eggs, unrefined or fortified and whole grain cereals and raw peanuts. Brewer's yeast tablets are particularly recommended. Plan to eat liver or kidney once or twice a week in the first weeks (have some slices of home-made liver pâté in the deep freeze for quick easy salad lunches).

Eat an egg, a portion of dark green leafy vegetables and two to three fruits daily. Have plenty to drink to prevent constipation and ensure enough for milk supply. Natural thirst should be quenched and not overlooked when you are busy. You need a lot of Vitamin C and iron for your own health after birth.

Eat a little polyunsaturated fats, preferably sunflower oil or soft margarine, and take 1 pint (575 ml) of milk (or as yogurt or cheese) daily if breast-feeding. *Eat every three to four hours yourself.* Six small meals daily, as during pregnancy, are best to prevent fatigue and post-natal depression, and those meals recommended for pregnancy are also most suitable after the birth of your child.

After six weeks check your weight. If you need to lose do this *slowly*; breast-feeding will help you. Move to a higher fibre diet, eat small meals at regular intervals. Reduce animal fats, sugar and refined cereals and bread. If you change to skimmed milk and cottage cheese take Vitamin D supplements to protect your bones and quality of milk, particularly in the winter months. Aim at only 1 lb (450 g) per week weight loss.

Foods to avoid

There is very little proper information on foods that a mother might eat and that might affect her baby adversely. It is believed that some proteins may pass to the milk unchanged. There are a very few highly sensitive babies who appear to show allergic reactions to large quantities of milk or egg in their mother's diet. If your totally breast-fed baby develops eczema (and this is rare), it may be worth considering reducing your intake of egg and/or milk to see if this helps. You should not consider dropping breast-feeding which is likely to make the condition worse. There is no proof that your eating certain foods will give your baby colic, but it is wise to choose decaffeinated coffee, for instance, as caffeine may pass into your milk.

Drugs to avoid

Alcohol does not enter the milk but a high intake can reduce the milk supply. One small drink may be beneficial in the early evening before a feed to help mother to relax.

Aspirin-based drugs are not recommended. They enter the milk and may cause aspirin allergy in baby to develop. Use Paracetamol in preference.

Antibiotics may cause penicillin allergy in baby later, may damage baby's teeth, and may cause anaemia. Always advise doctor that you are breast-feeding so that suitable antibiotics or other drugs are prescribed.

Antithyroid drugs, cortisone, steroids and epileptic drugs need careful monitoring. If you have to take long-term medication of any kind, seek doctor's advice before considering breast-feeding. It may be inadvisable.

Do not take any laxatives without consulting your doctor – they enter your milk. Eat a high fibre diet and take plenty of fluid if constipation is a problem. Take prunes and prune juice as a natural and safe laxative food.

If on the pill, low oestrogen doses are usually quite suitable if breast-feeding, although some doctors prefer other methods of contraception at this time. Mothers *fully* breast-feeding (with no bottles or solid foods) are unlikely to become pregnant in the first months but this is not considered completely safe.

Smoking is likely to reduce milk supply and nicotine will pass into your milk. Nevertheless your child's life and health are *less* at risk if you breast-feed rather than bottle-feed your baby. Do not allow people to smoke in the same room as infants and young children.

Sedatives, sleeping tablets and tranquillisers may affect baby in large doses, so check with your doctor. Taking these tablets can make you more prone to accidents, more aggressive and more at risk of baby battering. Accept all the support and help you can from family, friends and neighbours.

How to breast-feed

Breast-feeding does not come naturally to every mother, and the first few weeks especially are very much a learning period for both you *and* your baby. How to get yourself and your baby into a comfortable position for feeding, and your nipple in the best position in your baby's mouth is best demonstrated to you by the midwife in the first few days after birth. In the early days after you return home, you will probably need further advice and support to enable you to enjoy prolonged breast-feeding (see Appendix II).

There is no correlation between breast size and future success of breast-feeding. Whether you are flat-chested or large-busted, the breasts will develop and be able to produce milk. Both your baby's sucking efficiency and your own comfort can be much improved by ensuring your baby is properly positioned at the breast. For most mothers all, or nearly all, of the areola (darkened skin behind the nipple) will be in the baby's mouth so that he sucks on this area of the breast and not on the more tender nipple. Make sure your baby opens his mouth wide with his tongue forwards before tucking the nipple and breast well in. Ensure adequate support, using cushions if necessary.

To make the skin of the nipple stronger and less prone to cracking later, it is normal to wash the breast and nipple daily with soap and water and rub dry with a terry towel and massage in a little lanolin or similar hand, body or face cream to keep the skin elastic. Those with a very dry skin prone to cracking or to eczema, may find their skin generally improved by consuming 1 to 2 teaspoons of safflower oil daily. This will greatly increase your comfort when breast-feeding.

During the first weeks and months when only milk feeds are given it is a good idea to take the opportunity of putting your feet up. Make yourself very comfortable on a bed, sofa or large bean bag on the floor. Have your back well supported for comfort. In these early weeks you can pick up your baby and put him to the breast any time he is restless so that he can be satisfied and comforted.

Expect short frequent feeds in the first days as they are easier for your baby's stomach to digest and will reduce risks to you of uncomfortable engorgement when breasts are over-full and hard and sore. Feeding baby for only five to ten minutes on each side at short intervals (every two to three hours during the day) in the first ten to fourteen days, reduces these problems. Suckling time can thereafter be as long as your baby wants at the first breast and then the second breast can be offered if he is interested. Always start feeding on alternate breasts at each feed to maintain even supply.

To settle a restless baby, many mothers find best results may be had by feeding baby for about ten minutes on one side to satisfy his main hunger. Follow that by changing him, then allow as long on the second side as is needed to relax him and perhaps allow him to fall asleep so he can then be put in his cot with a minimum of disturbance.

Many mothers worry that they do not have enough milk. Even mothers with small breasts could provide enough milk for five babies simultaneously given time, so there is no reason why any mother of twins or triplets should feel the slightest concern about being unable to provide enough milk. And it is very easy to stimulate your supply of milk – just feed your baby more often and for a little longer for several days.

Topping up with a formula feed should only be used in an emergency if you have had a bad or very tiring day. This may give you a better night's sleep and then you can give yourself time to give much more regular feeds the following day to increase your own supply. Too frequent topping up with a bottle can be counter-productive as less milk will be drawn from the breasts and, lacking stimulation, they will gradually supply less and less.

At six weeks baby's appetite may quite suddenly

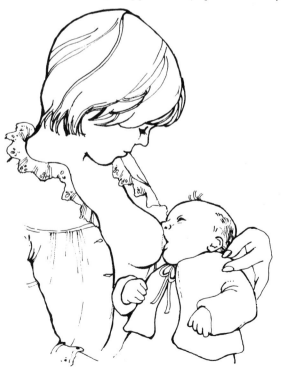

increase so increase number of feeds if necessary for a few days. Your breasts are now working much more efficiently and will rarely feel full, although able to provide a large supply. The milk now gradually increases in food value so an increase in quantity is not so important. Your baby will soon last longer between feeds. If there is a later sudden demand for more food, common at three to four months, increase the number of feeds rather than turning too early to solid feeding. Milk alone provides enough food for five to six months.

To feed your own baby until seven months old, when mixed feeding is well established, is a tremendous advantage to his health and welfare. There is no reason why a child should not continue with a breast-feed at bedtime or during times of illness or stress until well after his first year. It is wise to gradually tail off breast-feeding when you are expecting another baby but there are no firm rules that have to be followed. The decision should be that of mother and baby alone.

Breast-feeding problems

Nearly every mother should be able to enjoy breast-feeding for many months. Always ask for help quickly if you are worried. Help is available twenty-four hours a day if it is needed (see Appendix II).

Do not give up breast-feeding if your baby is having problems, or start on solid feeding too early. This is never the answer to difficulties for a baby under four months. Try your doctor, health visitor, or a breast-feeding counsellor from La Lèche League or the National Childbirth Trust – whoever inspires the most confidence. If you feel something is wrong with your baby's health contact your doctor promptly.

Breast-feeding and illness

Mothers with whooping cough or TB are usually the only ones who are recommended to discontinue feeding because of infection. If you have to go into hospital for any condition it is often possible to take your baby in with you so do make enquiries and seek medical advice before automatically abandoning feeding your baby. It may be possible to express a little milk regularly to keep your supply going; and your hospital may be able to supply breast milk from their milk bank which is preferable to switching to cow's milk formula.

Let-down reflex

This is the sensation you may feel in the breasts when you think of your baby, hear him cry or begin to suckle him, caused by the natural movement of the milk towards the nipple. When you are tired or tense, though, the milk may not be let down through the nipple as quickly, so a little patience is needed. Try to make yourself much more comfortable while feeding. Put your feet up with a drink, snack, music or magazines, and give yourself and baby plenty of time.

Mastitis

This is an infection in the breast which can cause great discomfort. You may have a fever with a reddened patch of inflammation on the breast. Use warm, not cold, compresses on breasts and seek medical help very quickly so proper treatment can be given without delay. Breast-feeding can and should be continued, and you should feed baby more often for your greater comfort.

Cracked nipples

Dry nipple well and rub in a little salad oil just after feeding baby. Pure lanolin is best if nipples are sore, but mineral oils should never be used. Keep nipples dry between feeds, and do not use plastic liners in bra – absorbent tissue is much better. Use a nursing bra with flaps that drop down and expose nipples to air (if possible in the sun) to dry and improve the skin. Some mothers who have a severe problem with nipples tuck a pair of plastic tea strainers in the bra (cut the plastic handles off first!) which protect sore nipples well and allow them to stay dry. Ensure your baby is sucking on the breast not your nipples for your comfort. Seek medical help quickly if they are becoming really painful.

Returning to work

This should be delayed as long as possible if you wish to continue breast-feeding. To combine a day's work with breast-feeding is not very easy; unlike the cow who supplies milk when milked twice a day, the human mother is designed as a continuous or very frequent feeder to maintain a good milk supply. A gap of six to eight hours between feeds during the day will diminish her supply but some mothers are happy to express milk during working hours to store in a fridge (label carefully or it could end up in someone's coffee!). Part-time work when only the odd bottle-feed need be given presents no problems.

New views on breast-feeding

During the last few years there has been a great increase in the use of breast milk for the feeding of premature infants. The milk may be provided by the natural mother but frequently comes from the breast milk bank reserves held by some hospitals for frail infants who might be at greater risk if a modified cow's milk is given. Hospitals will welcome surplus breast milk for their special care units.

In previous centuries it used to be common practice for wealthy mothers to employ a wet nurse for their infants. This has been viewed with horror by many who have turned to bottle-feeding in the past and present. Nevertheless the move to breast milk banks show that this practice *does* still have a place in the modern world.

Communal breast-feeding

Amongst close friends and sisters there have been cases where much help and support has been given by a confident mother successfully breast-feeding her own baby, giving an occasional feed to a baby whose mother is having difficulties. If a mother's milk supply is poor because of insufficient stimulation from her own baby she may find this difficulty eased by putting a strong sucking child to her breast several times over a period of a few days to improve her supply.

Equally, a generous supply to her own baby may help *him* get the hang of efficient suckling. Other mothers may use this system to breast-feed when baby-sitting for friends if their own milk supply is good. Mothers wishing to return to work may find a friend willing to feed her baby during working hours.

Breast-feeding adopted babies

Even a woman who has never had a baby is able to breast-feed if she is determined to try, and a growing number of mothers of adopted babies are doing so. It was not uncommon in many backward countries where maternal mortality was high and a sister, aunt or grandmother had to look after the baby.

Breast-feeding gives an added bonding of mother and baby even if only partially successful. Supplementary feeds will have to be given so that the baby remains keen to suckle at the breast even before a milk supply becomes established – which will come gradually after a few days and increase over the next weeks. One aid to mothers attempting to feed adopted babies is the Lact-Aid (contact La Lèche League). This is a small bag which hangs round the mother's neck containing milk. It has a fine tube that is placed in the baby's mouth to suck, along with the nipple, which will stimulate the breasts to produce milk at the same time as gratifying his hunger. Mothers should be prepared to supplement the milk feed of their baby even when breast feeding

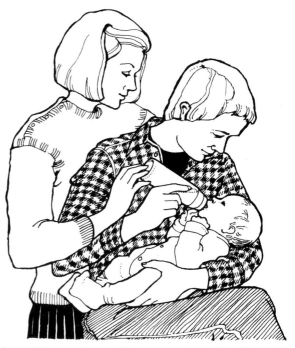

is established since milk may not be as plentiful as in a mother who has given birth. Seek advice from a breast-feeding councillor who will encourage your endeavours.

Formula bottle-feeding

Great improvements have been made in recent years in the quality of milk formulae for bottle-feeding. Research has proved that doorstep cow's milk is *not* suitable for a baby until after six months, and so babies should be given one of the specially formulated milks to ensure their good health. Although not every mother can breast-feed with comfort or pleasure – and in a few cases medical reasons make it inadvisable – every mother wants to find the best possible alternative to ensure her baby has a good start in life.

The most important thing, apart from the right formula, is to ensure that the bottle-fed baby is held as lovingly by his mother, father or regular childminder as the breast-fed baby. During the early weeks especially, he should not be handed round with his bottle from one apparent stranger to another, but should be fed regularly by the same two people in order that he may develop a bond with them.

Choosing the formula

It is very difficult to decide which milk you should buy for your baby. Health visitors are not allowed to name and recommend their favourite brands but, in practice, those that they believe are the most suitable for you to use are likely in many areas to be those that they offer cheaply at their baby clinics. You will save a little on each packet, and you will eventually use about two packets per week. While at the clinic you can also buy cheap vitamin supplements and have your baby checked.

For most babies, you should be looking for a baby milk formula that most closely resembles human milk. An exact copy is impossible but many modifications can now be made to produce milk which is similar. This will reduce some of the disadvantages of bottle-feeding, the major one of which is that antibodies (to help fight infections) cannot be added to formula milk. It is for this reason that all mothers should, if possible, try to give their babies colostrum, which comes into the breast before the milk and is so rich in protective factors. This lasts for five days and is a great advantage to their baby even if they have no intention of continuing to breast-feed.

Choose a formula in which the sodium level is low (breast milk only contains 15 mg per 3½ fl. oz or 100 ml). Those that are in the region of 15–20 mg are preferable in the first weeks. All baby milk formulae are now well below the sodium level of cow's milk to reduce the risk of dehydration.

Milk formula is available with milk fat partly reduced and replaced with vegetable oil (often safflower oil) so that the fatty acids more closely resemble human milk. The level of linoleic fatty acids is much higher in breast than cow's milk and is required for proper growth. The vegetable oils are high in unsaturated fatty acids so may be better for long-term health. These milks are thus preferable.

Protein level should be only a little above that of breast milk. This is to allow for the proportions of the essential amino acids (of which protein is made) being supplied in sufficient quantity. Cow's milk and human milk vary in the proportion of these so this will allow for variation. The proportion of casein to the soluble whey protein in human milk is different from cow's milk (formula containing whey is more readily digested).

All milks are suitably fortified with minerals and vitamins. The milks which most closely resemble breast milk and are therefore likely to be the best choice are:
Gold Cap (SMA, S26), *Osterfeed* (Farley), *Premium* (Cow and Gate).

It has been noted that the regurgitation of infants fed Osterfeed smells more like that of breast milk than other formula milk. A very small advantage, but could indicate it is in some way closer to breast milk.

Having chosen a milk that suits your baby there is no need to change to a different feed. If your baby seems very hungry before three to four months it is an indication that he needs either a larger bottle at each feed or, more likely, *more* day-time feeds. Try and work in another morning or afternoon feed to satisfy his hunger rather than presuming he needs a different milk or mixed feeding. It may be that he is getting his feed too fast and that it is lack of sucking time which is making him dissatisfied, especially if he is unhappy after a larger but rather quick feed.

The three powdered formula milks recommended for babies and some other formulae are available as a ready-to-feed milk in disposable bottles. In practice they are only widely used in hospitals to save expensive time and space for the making up of sterile feeds. They are not so economically viable at home but could be very useful for travelling or camping. They are vacuum-packed, usually in two sizes, and can be stored and used at room (car or caravan) temperature. No refrigerator is necessary. Ask at your local chemist for details and availability, and check whether you can order them if not in stock.

A paediatrician will advise you if your baby is premature or has a particular digestive problem and requires a specially modified milk.

If your baby has been or is ill your doctor or health visitor will advise you if a change of milk is desirable. Sometimes after gastroenteritis a milk lower in lactose – Milumil or Ostermilk complete formula – may be more easily digested for a period.

Bottles

These may be of glass or plastic. The latter tend to discolour with age, especially when used for blackcurrant juice (although this does not mean they are unsuitable to use). Glass may be broken if dropped so choose which you feel will suit you best: your baby won't know the difference. There is little advantage between the different traditional designs of bottles, and the cheapest will be in sets of three from large chain baby stores and chemists.

You may prefer to buy four to six bottles plus sterilising unit and lidded jug in a complete set. Note that some sterilising units do not come with bottles or jugs, and are therefore not such a good buy. In fact the units are not essential as a 1 gallon (4.5 litre)

Making Up Powdered Milk Formulae

Milk formulae are usually sold as powders to be mixed with warm boiled water according to the manufacturers' instructions. Follow them carefully.

1. Water from the cold tap should be used. *Never* use water from the hot tap, and never use water which has passed through a water softener. Substances used in the softening of water contain sodium and are not very suitable for mixing with feeds when making up bottles. In your home ensure that water going to the cold tap in the kitchen by-passes your home water softener for your whole family's health.

2. To ensure tap water is fresh, wait until after breakfast to prepare feeds when plenty of water will have been run through the household pipes.

3. Empty kettle completely before filling with fresh water – do not boil water twice or keep topping the kettle up as it alters the mineral concentration.

4. Cool water in kettle, sterilised covered jug or sterile bottles until hand-hot.

5. Measure water very accurately and add to the warm water one level scoop (as supplied by the brand of milk you are using) per 1 fl. oz (25 ml) water or as indicated on packet. Level scoop using clean straight-edged knife. **Do not** pack down first. Shake bottle before inserting teat, or stir well.

According to your own convenience, you can either make each individual feed as you want it (so you need at least two bottles), which is a little time-consuming, or you can prepare enough feed to last up to twenty-four hours, to be stored in the refrigerator. One way of doing this is to make in a jug with a lid that you can sterilise. You also need at least two bottles to sterilise and fill from jug as needed. This is a very flexible method if you do not know how much or many feeds your baby may need. You could also make up about twenty-four hours' supply directly in the bottles to store in the fridge. You will need six bottles.

Allow each day 2½ fl. oz (75 ml) milk per 1 lb (500 g) of baby's weight, and divide between number of feeds given in twenty-four hours. As an example, if the baby is on five feeds a day:

Allow at each feed:
1 fl. oz (30 ml) per 2 lb (1 kg) of baby's weight
Therefore:
5 fl. oz (150 ml) for a 10 lb (5 kg) baby
6 fl. oz (175 ml) for a 12 lb (6 kg) baby
This is only a guide, as appetites vary considerably as they do in children and adults.

plastic ice cream carton or similar can be used, but remember that all items must be submerged – including teats which tend to float if not weighted down by jam jar or plastic grid.

Bottles with sterile liners

You will require only one bottle which is very cheap plus one to two of the specially designed teats which are about the price of the traditional bottles. Packs of disposable sterile liners are used with these. It will cost about double the normal cost of sterilising traditional bottles daily with sterilising tablets and a little more than using one of the hyperchlorite solutions for babies' bottles. This extra cost can be partly offset by a reduced initial outlay on equipment, but if you use the same equipment for more than one baby the traditional bottle will be cheaper. One advantage of these bottles with liners is that air is not sucked in with the milk, nor does baby have to stop feeding for air to replace milk sucked out of the conventional bottle since the inner lining collapses as the baby feeds. A further advantage of this bottle is that the teat is designed like a nipple on a breast so that it seems more like breast feeding to the baby.

Teats

Mothers tend to speed feeds up for their own convenience by using a large nipple hole or holes in teats but this is not good for your baby. His teeth and jaw formation will suffer through lack of suckling and will result in him being almost force-fed with gushing milk as he fulfils his natural desire to suck.

The orthodontic teat (available from the National Childbirth Trust, if not in your local shops) should be used by all new babies on any standard bottles in the hope that this will minimise the disadvantage of bottle-feeding on the development of the jaw and teeth. Where parents and other members of the family tend to have crowded, thus crooked, teeth it is most important that an effort is made to try to prevent this tendency at the earliest possible stage. Changing from the conventional to the orthodontic teat later is likely to be unpopular with your baby.

All teats should have one to three holes off-centre on the nipple. The breast does not have one large hole in the centre, and if this is all there is in a teat it may cause a gush of milk at the back of a baby's throat and make him gag if he sucks hard.

If using the bottles with disposable liners, do use the teat designed for the new baby for under six months, not that designed for the older baby which will have a larger nipple. Order these from your chemist if they do not have them in stock.

Sterilising

Before sterilisation can be properly achieved bottles must be thoroughly cleaned. Use ordinary washing-up liquid and a bottle brush. Stubborn milk scum on teats can be rubbed off both inside and outside with salt. Rinse all items well under running water before sterilising. Follow instructions with chosen sterilising method carefully.

Sterilising tablets

These are cheapest bought in large quantities from chainstore chemists or baby stores. They are very convenient to use and the quickest (about half an hour) method of sterilisation.

Hyperchlorite solutions

These are much more expensive, and may take three times as long.

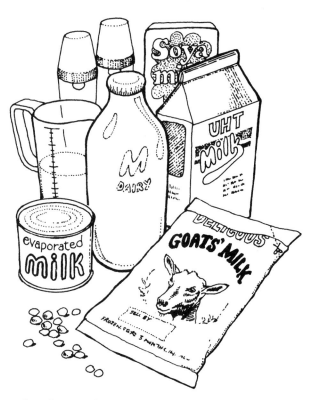

Alternative milks and other drinks

For most babies formula or breast milk will be the most suitable until seven months, and can be continued until one year. But there will be some with special requirements.

Do not suddenly change from breast to a high sodium milk, nor quickly from a low sodium baby milk to doorstep cow's milk. In some babies the sudden increase in sodium can cause fast weight gain and water retention while the kidneys become accustomed to disposing of extra sodium content. If a sudden change from breast milk has to be undertaken choose the low sodium milks like Gold Cap, Osterfeed or Premium. (Choose a bottle with the new orthodontic teat for preference when moving from breast to bottle, which is likely to be the most acceptable for your baby.)

Doorstep cow's milk

Between six and eight months most babies are moved *slowly* to doorstep milk. Your baby clinic will usually advise you when this is suitable for your baby. It is also wise to wait until after a good range of solid foods have been tried on your baby (see next chapter). If you make this move at the beginning of solid feeding, you may be unable to identify the cause of any stomach upset or rashes.

Doorstep milk should never be given to a baby under six months without the addition of water as the sodium and protein content are much too high for a small baby. Doorstep milk is not recommended as a regular feed before six months. It requires a number of modifications and fortifications to bring the baby's feed closer to that of a mother's natural milk and this is important for the baby's short- and long-term health and safety.

Silver top pasteurised or *semi-skimmed* pasteurised milks should be chosen, not the gold- or green-topped high-fat milks. *Red/silver topped* homogenised (fat finely dispersed) milk is also suitable, as is *UHT (Ultra Heat Treated) Long Life full cream milk*, but do *not* use the skimmed milks which lack the fatty acids and Vitamins A and D needed by growing babies and children. (These are British Milk Marketing Board colour coding.)

These four varieties of milk are considered safe and suitable for most infants over six to seven months, immediately they are opened. All can be rapidly affected by bacteria if not kept in perfect condition, which means they *must* be kept refrigerated, either in the original container or transferred to a sterilised covered jug or feeding bottle and used the same day.

In practice many health visitors still feel happier to recommend that milk is boiled and then poured straight into sterile feeding bottles or sterile covered jug specially for baby, to reduce the risk of contamination that could occur after milk bottles are casually opened and left about. Some health visitors may feel they achieve a better health record for infants under their care if they advise all mothers to boil milk until twelve months.

A further advantage in either boiling the different pasteurised milks first, or using UHT full cream milk, or evaporated milk – when correctly diluted – is that the high temperatures that each is subjected to alters the protein fat molecules in the milk making them a little easier to digest. The flavour and texture of each is slightly different, and your baby may have a preference, but nutritionally they are all suitable.

Goat's milk

It is advised to boil this milk for all children as hygiene standards from suppliers vary. The supply of goat's milk may not be continuous throughout the year so check with your supplier. The milk may be frozen but this can cause a stronger flavour to develop.

Goat's milk (boiled) is suitable from six to seven months or when a move to doorstep cow's milk has been recommended. It is lower than cow's milk in Vitamins A, D and C, as well as folic acid and Vitamin B_{12}. Give the normal supplement of Vitamins A, D and C daily and ensure that folic acid and B_{12} are adequate in the diet by giving liver or kidney once or twice a week, eggs and green vegetables regularly, or by giving an artificial supplement of B_{12} and folic acid. Goat's milk is lower in sodium than cow's milk, an advantage to the young. It may reduce allergic conditions, so is worth trying if your baby has problems.

Goat's milk should always be modified as below for infants under six to seven months.

To make 1 pint boil together	To make 1000 ml boil together
16 fl. oz goat's milk	800 ml goat's milk
4 fl. oz water	200 ml water
¾ oz sugar	35 g sugar

Soya bean milk

Powdered or liquid soya milk is available at health-food shops and some chemists. Make up according to manufacturers' instructions. For babies over six to seven months and children use with a good normal diet and give fish regularly (soya milk may be low in iodine). Give normal supplements of Vitamins A, D and C. Soya milk is otherwise similar in nutritional value to cow's milk.

For babies, especially those under six to seven months, check manufacturers' instructions relating to infant feeding or seek medical advice. Appropriate soya milk can be given from birth for infants with allergic problems, and it is probably wise to give this milk under medical supervision.

Evaporated milk

Suitable for infants after six to seven months when doorstep cow's milk is recommended. Reconstitute as directed: 1½ parts water to 1 part evaporated milk. (Please note that US evaporated milk has a different concentration.) For babies under six months evaporated milk is not normally now recommended, as modern baby formulae are superior nutritionally.

Condensed milk is *not* recommended for infants or children of any age – it's far too high in sugar.

Dried milk

Dried milks designed for general consumption are not like baby milks which are modified and elaborately fortified. They are not suitable for babies during the period when milk is the major part of the diet. In an emergency they could be used after seven to nine months, but fresh or whole UHT milk should always be chosen in preference throughout childhood as the main source of milk when fortified baby milks are phased out, or breast-feeding ceases (if after seven months).

Special milks for problem babies

A wide range of 'milks' are made for a variety of digestive disorders and these are available on your doctor's recommendation for use when breast milk or normal baby milks are not considered ideal.

Water

Tap water should be boiled until a baby is six to seven months, longer in some areas. It is often convenient to pour some boiled water into a sterile bottle at the beginning of the day. Cool then chill. If baby is thirsty this can be given cold, or a little freshly boiled water may be added to it to warm it so that you do not have to wait for a boiling drink to cool for a screaming baby.

Your health visitor can advise on the safety of water in your area. To reduce the risk of contamination from the water pipes run half a sinkful of water off before using for baby.

Fruit drinks

The best nutritional value lies in fresh squeezed citrus fruits, the juice of which contains many trace elements of value in the diet. It should be given by spoon or mug not bottle so that useful elements do not have to be strained out.

With a suitable extractor, vegetable juices high in Vitamin C may be made at home from cauliflower, cabbage, turnips, and green beans. To make fresh vegetable juices without an extractor, purée half a cup chopped vegetables with one cup of cool boiled water in an electric processor or blender. When fine press through a sieve to strain and separate from pulp. All other fruits and vegetables have only a low level of Vitamin C.

Guide to Fruit Juices

If you buy commercial fruit juices choose:

- Cartons of pasteurised unsweetened fruit juice without additives. Some cartons can be ordered through the milkman.
- Tins of unsweetened fruit juices, without additives, as well as tomato juice.
- Jars of unsweetened fruit juices.
- Frozen concentrated fruit juices (particularly economical and compact when shopping).

Do not buy sweetened powdered breakfast drinks like Apeel. Commercial sweetened baby juices are only necessary if you cannot find an alternative that suits your baby. Rosehip is unlikely to cause an allergic conditions.

The following all provide 40–50 mg of Vitamin C.

- 3–3½ fl. oz (90–100 ml) fresh squeezed citrus juice. Best used in 3–4 days.
- 4 fl. oz (115 ml) pasteurised orange and grapefruit juice from cartons. Best used in 3–4 days.
- 4 fl. oz (115 ml) jar or canned orange, grapefruit juice. Best used in 2–3 days.
- 4 fl. oz (115 ml) reconstituted frozen citrus juice (see below). Best used in 3–4 days.
- 6 fl. oz (175 ml) canned tomato juice. Best used in 2–3 days.
- 3–6 fl. oz (90–175 ml) home-made vegetable juice. Best used same day.

Frozen citrus juice – preferably orange – should be reconstituted with *cold boiled* water for babies if storing for three to four days in refrigerator. For both babies and children it is often preferable to dilute juices with water; frozen juices can be mixed with up to nine parts water, the others equal parts water and juice. Allow for this when estimating Vitamin C value which is based on recommended reconstitution on carton. Some juices are very acid and can upset a baby's stomach. If this is a problem choose fresh orange diluted one part juice to three parts cold boiled water, or use vegetable juices or commercial baby juices until about five to seven months.

Commercial baby juices are all made with a sweet syrup base. Glucose, not sucrose, is now used to lessen the risk of damage to teeth. They should be given well diluted with about 2–3 fl. oz (60–90 ml) cooled boiled water and given at a convenient time.

Never heat juices or the Vitamin C will be destroyed. Apple, pineapple and fruit juices other than citrus, guava and tomato, are low in Vitamin C so should not be used as the daily source. They are, nevertheless, a good drink. Carrot, apricot, peach and mango juices are very high in Vitamin A but not C.

If a cup is to be used for a baby choose one with two handles and open lip spout, not a mug with a small-holed spout which the child will suck. This will train them to use an adult cup or mug, which is also sipped not sucked.

Feeding times

A much more relaxed view is now held about how often a baby should be fed. Many now believe he should be picked up any time he is fretful, especially if it is some time since he has had a meal (two hours or more), and he is very young. Breast-feeding offers the most flexible method at first. A quick 'nip' when he is restless often helps a baby to relax and sleep. It will not always be necessary to change his nappy at every feed if there is a relatively short gap since his last change.

Bottle-fed babies usually need feeding less often than breast-fed. The milk takes longer to digest, being less perfectly designed for the infant's stomach, so the feeling of hunger is slower to return. Gaps usually start at two and a half to four and a half hours for a breast-fed baby, three to five hours for a bottle-fed, so while three and a half to four hours is a rough guide it is not something to do by the clock.

Family life-style will to some extent infringe on your baby's demands for food. It may be that you will have to wake him for a feed or make him last a little longer if his demands clash with those of the family who have perhaps trains and buses to catch and other schedules to meet. Where possible anticipate your baby's needs if you think he will want feeding at an inconvenient time, and feed him early. It is very wearing for everyone, listening to a hungry baby cry.

Babies who learn from an early age that they have to become quite frantic screaming for their basic needs to be met, will not develop happy and contented dispositions, and many develop into very

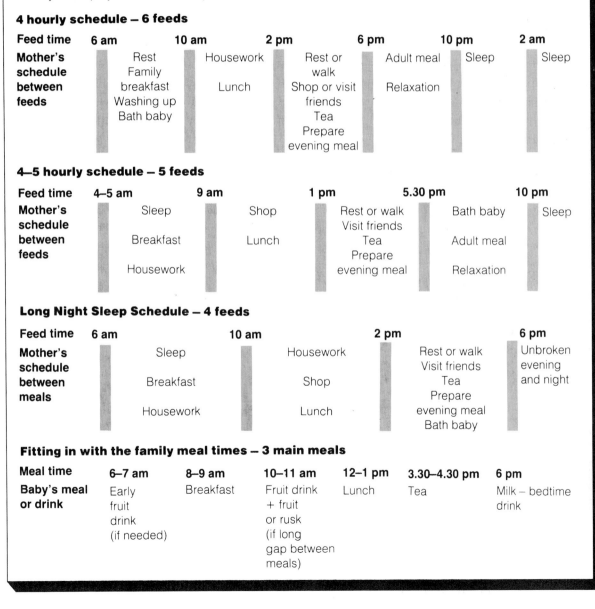

Feeding schedules

Do not use these with a stop watch in hand, as most babies will not conveniently slot into them for long. Nevertheless they do provide a useful framework of a day's plan, and without a little overall organisation the day can slip by with little but baby minding and a few chores achieved.

4 hourly schedule — 6 feeds

Feed time	6 am	10 am	2 pm	6 pm	10 pm	2 am
Mother's schedule between feeds	Rest Family breakfast Washing up Bath baby	Housework Lunch	Rest or walk Shop or visit friends Tea Prepare evening meal	Adult meal Relaxation	Sleep	Sleep

4—5 hourly schedule — 5 feeds

Feed time	4–5 am	9 am	1 pm	5.30 pm	10 pm
Mother's schedule between feeds	Sleep Breakfast Housework	Shop Lunch	Rest or walk Visit friends Tea Prepare evening meal	Bath baby Adult meal Relaxation	Sleep

Long Night Sleep Schedule — 4 feeds

Feed time	6 am	10 am	2 pm	6 pm
Mother's schedule between meals	Sleep Breakfast Housework	Housework Shop Lunch	Rest or walk Visit friends Tea Prepare evening meal Bath baby	Unbroken evening and night

Fitting in with the family meal times — 3 main meals

Meal time	6–7 am	8–9 am	10–11 am	12–1 pm	3.30–4.30 pm	6 pm
Baby's meal or drink	Early fruit drink (if needed)	Breakfast	Fruit drink + fruit or rusk (if long gap between meals)	Lunch	Tea	Milk – bedtime drink

Meal schedules from birth through childhood

Early Morning	Morning	Middle of Day	Afternoon	Evening

1—4 months

Breast or bottle feed	Breast or bottle feed	Breast or bottle feed	Breast or bottle feed	Breast or bottle feed + night feed if needed

4—5 months

Breast or bottle feed	Breast or bottle feed 1–2 tsp rice	1 tbsp stewed veg. Breast or bottle feed	1–2 tsp fruit purée Breast or bottle feed	Breast or bottle feed (if baby wakes)

5—6 months

Breast or bottle feed	½ cup rice cereal and fruit purée Breast or bottle feed	1–2 tbsp veg. purée + 1 tbsp lamb, chicken, or liver Milk or bottle feed	Egg, milk, or cheese or fruit purée Breast or bottle feed	Breast or bottle feed (if baby wakes)

Fruit juice from 6 weeks

6—8 months

On Waking	Breakfast 8—9 am	Lunch 12—1 pm	Tea 3.30—5 pm	Bedtime 6—7 pm
Fruit juice	½ cup high protein/ mixed baby cereal (not rice) or cooked breakfast – soft boiled egg, or grilled chopped bacon and tomato, with rusk or toast Breast or cup of milk	Meat, fish, poultry or ground nuts or pulses + pasta, rice or potato, + vegetables. Finger foods + milk or yogurt dessert with fruit juice, or fruit with small milk drink	Veg. or fruit dish + cheese, egg, rusk or bread Finger foods + breast or cup of milk	Breast, bottle or cup of milk

8 months to 11 years

On Waking	Breakfast	Elevenses	Lunch	Tea	Bedtime
Fruit juice (or give fruit at breakfast)	Baby or suitable breakfast cereal + cooked breakfast if wished	Fruit or milk drink + fruit if required	Meat, poultry, fish, nut or pulses + vegetables + potato, rice or pasta + fruit or milk dessert + fruit juice or water	Cheese, egg, nut or pulses + vegetables + fruit + bread + milk	Milk drink

aggressively demanding people. You *cannot* spoil a baby by picking him up to feed or comfort him as soon as he cries. Learning to be disciplined and considerate of others is part of the education of a child, *not* of a new baby.

Night feeds

Many mothers worry about how to get a baby to understand you want him to sleep through the night without regular feeds. This is solved comparatively easily by making the atmosphere of the night feeds quite different from the day right from the start. Sing, talk and play with your baby at the day-time feeds in a well-lit room, then at night keep the room as dark as possible, using just a small torch or night-light so you can see what you are doing. Do not play with your baby, sing or talk, but be very quiet. Trying to fill babies up in the evening and giving solid foods is not the answer to the problem of infants who need regular feeds through the night for a protracted period. Some babies need night-time feeds well beyond the six-week to three-month period we consider average, and it is less wearing and frustrating to accept this than to try and fight the problem.

As your baby grows and manages to last longer between feeds, do not allow this to extend to four and a half to five hours during the day, but lift him to feed after about four hours whenever possible, so that the five meals from 4 or 6 o'clock in the morning until your last feed as you go to bed at night stay roughly at the same time. You can reasonably hope that the 2 am feed will gradually slide to merge with just one early-morning feed.

Once the middle of the night feed is dropped you and your baby can work towards dropping either the early-morning feed or the late-night feed, depending on what suits you both. If you are late getting up in the morning you may choose to continue to wake and feed your baby as you go to bed, rather than risk being disturbed too early. On the other hand, your child may have a mind of his own about which suits him, so be prepared to be flexible.

For a rough schedule of what your days and nights might be like, look at the charts on the previous pages. But you must be flexible. Few weeks will ever be the same and just when he has developed one pattern of sleep, feed and play he will grow into the next. Try to break up your other daily activities into short periods; for example, do not plan to clean the whole house in one go. By having short activities your day will not be too disrupted by breaking off what you are doing to meet your baby's needs, and jobs you are planning to do can be slipped in just as easily before or after a feed.

Chapter Four
From weaning to family meals

It is surprising how quickly babies can bridge the gap between tasting food for the first time and eating much of the food you are giving the whole family. Judging by the shelves of baby foods in chemists' shops and supermarkets, one could be forgiven for thinking babies eat nothing but that stuff for years. In fact many never touch any of these prepared foods, although a few are sometimes useful.

Views on when to give solid foods to babies have changed remarkably in the past fifteen years. At one time very early solid feeding during the first six weeks was condoned, but the many problems resultant on this practice and our better understanding of nutrition, have produced quite different views.

1. Remember that your baby's digestive system is not fully developed at birth, and is designed to take only milk, not a wide range of foods.

2. Never start mixed feeding under four months. If your baby seems hungry and restless give more milk at feeds, longer sucking time, or more milk feeds per day. Check also that he is not thirsty.

3. Only consider solid feeds when birth weight doubles, when baby weighs over 15 lb (6.5–7 kg), when he takes 35 fl. oz (1 litre) milk daily, when his weight increase slows significantly, or when your doctor or clinic recommend it.

4. Don't be tempted to start mixed feeding early because all your friends do, or they say their babies always sleep through the night, or never cry or only need three feeds a day. Babies just *are* different, and filling them with food will not alter this. If you have problems with your baby seek *professional* advice.

Food supplements for infants and children

Five drops daily, or as directed, of the mixed vitamin supplement A, D and C should be taken until five years, unless appetite for a wide variety of foods is good. These are of particular value during the winter months; for children who eat few vegetables or who have a poor appetite; for children who live in high-rise flats, cities and industrial areas; and for children with dark skins. They may be continued until eleven years, but a full dose will not be required if your chosen breakfast cereal is reinforced with a high level of Vitamins A and D. Doses of A, D and C may be preferred as tablets (like mini-Smarties), but beware of giving to children under five years who will not appreciate the danger of taking overdoses.

Fluoride undoubtedly helps to harden growing teeth, protecting them against decay, and you should consult your dentist and doctor before using. There is, however, some concern as to whether it is good for general health, especially of young babies. Fluoride can be painted directly onto the teeth, if preferred, and in some areas it is free for all children under the age of sixteen when their permanent teeth develop.

Four to six months

For most babies the period between four and six months can be used to gradually accustom them to different tastes and textures in their mouths; to gradually train them in the new skill of coping with a spoon, 'solid' foods and swallowing solids. By six months babies do definitely need more than milk and fruit juice can supply. They need more iron particularly, and a wider range of nutrients. But they still need milk, and no other food can supply the protein, calcium and phosphorus in such ideal proportions for the growth of skull and development of brain.

Weaning

1. Start mixed feeding very slowly, testing each food carefully before moving to the next to make sure they suit your baby (see Chapter Nine on allergies).

2. Continue to breast-feed or bottle-feed, with the same type of milk so that there is no confusion between a new food or a new milk causing upset.

3. Offer solid food at first only when your baby is fairly hungry and in a good mood, and you are relaxed and not rushed.

4. Use a very small spoon or spatula (plastic coffee spoons are ideal), and offer only 1 spoonful at first.

5. Make food fairly soft and wet; it will frighten him if it is too tacky and sticks to the roof of his mouth.

6. Give baby most of his normal milk feed *before* offering a little food to suck off the spoon. If he is relaxed and fairly satisfied first he will be more amenable to change.

7. Do not shovel food in then try and wash it down with his milk feed; it will only make him gag. Never urge him to finish up all the food you have prepared, or the entire contents of a tin or jar.

8. Do not add cereal to his bottle feed; it leads to overweight.

9. Make yourself comfortable and protect your clothes and those of baby with bib, towel or tissues; you will then be more relaxed! Smile and be cheerful; your baby will be aware if you are tense or anxious.

10. Feed your baby in your arms in your normal feeding position, and only move to a slanted chair for solid feeds when baby is really enjoying his feed and nearly ready to move to a high chair.

11. Do not be surprised if your baby shows interest in solid food only a few times per week at first. Offer only a few tastes at the end of the feed until he shows an interest in a variety of foods. Do not reduce his intake of milk at this time, or worry if he goes off solid foods for a while.

12. Do not give solid food twice a day until 1–2 tablespoons of food are being taken once each day, then introduce a second solid feed at another convenient time. A mixed feed at 10 pm helps some babies to sleep longer at night, but this is certainly not true of all.

Established mixed feeding

In their sixth month most babies will be enjoying two to three meals a day, and will take between 1 and 2 tablespoons of mixed food at each. Up until this time food should be given *after* most of the milk feed so that the appetite for milk is not diminished (milk is still the most important food). But now, when he really welcomes solid foods, baby may be offered these *before* the breast or bottle, but it is still important not to give so much solid food that the milk consumption drops, as alternative foods given may have less food value than milk.

During the period from the start of mixed feeding until a varied diet is well established the consumption of milk and milk protein, minerals and vitamins is vital not just for the growing bones and teeth but for the growing skull and brain. If the baby's nutrition is inadequate during this time he will not reach his full intellectual potential; no amount of proteins, vitamins and minerals later on in life will make up for the damage done during this period. 1½–1¾ pints (850 ml–1 litre) of milk is a good guide for the requirements of babies of this age. Most purées will be only a poor substitute if the milk intake is allowed to drop.

This is the main reason for discouraging the practice of giving cereals and other foods in any quantity under six months. Large quantities of solid foods before and at this time are unlikely to provide the precise nutrients required for this important

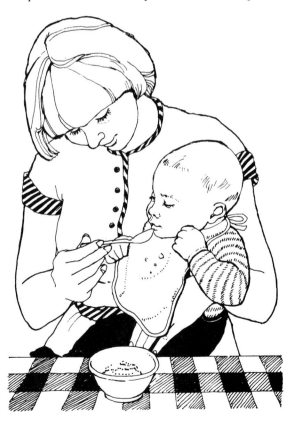

Foods to avoid

Foods which Carry Most Risk of Allergy

Gluten   In wheat, barley and sometimes oats.

Eggs   The whites especially should be given well cooked. Egg yolks should be given first.

Cow's milk   Also cheese and yogurt. Give modified formula milk only.

Fish   Especially shellfish.

Chocolate and cocoa   Use other flavourings, like carob.

Some fruits   Citrus fruits and strawberries can cause allergies. Orange juice is widely used for small babies but rosehip and blackcurrant are good alternatives for those with family history of citrus fruit allergy.

Mushrooms   Reaction in a very few people is severe, so they are not recommended early.

Chemical additions   Colour and flavourings etc. should be avoided wherever possible.

Foods which Carry Risk of Contamination

Bacteria   Bought cold meats, meat pies, sausages – avoid all of these at first; also cheese and minced meat in unhygienic conditions. Cook mince on day of purchase.

Food poisoning   Poultry must be well thawed and thoroughly cooked.

Lead or food poisoning   Shellfish, oily fish, tinned fish.

Badly stored   Badly frozen products may have lost food value or be contaminated. New potatoes turning green (store in the dark). Wash all fruit and vegetables before preparation.

Foods Difficult to Digest

Pips and seeds   In berries, currants, cooked tomato (but not raw – the jelly round these seeds acts as a lubricant).

Skins   Of dried fruit, grapes, tomatoes.

Cooked cheese   Boiling in sauces etc. toughens the protein.

Fats and oils   In fried and fatty foods: pastries, fatty minced meat, oily fish.

Salt   Only small quantity needed – difficult for baby under eight months to excrete excess.

Green vegetables   Especially likely to cause wind if *overcooked*.

Dried pulses   Lentils, beans, etc. likely to cause wind, so give in small quantities only at first.

Foods which do not Contribute to Nutritional Needs

Sugar   Calories only

Modified starches   Calories mainly and mask poor quality of commercial purées.

Squash drinks   Calories, chemicals and no nutritional value.

Refined cereals   Those highly refined for normal cooking are of little value to a baby and should be used sparingly – ground and flaked rice, cornflour, tapioca, sago, etc.

development, and invariably mean the milk consumption is substantially lessened. However small quantities will help a baby learn to become accustomed to a variety of foods and can provide additional supplements of nutrients such as iron that are comparatively lacking in milk.

Only 1 teaspoon of solids was offered at first during the weaning stage; this can gradually be increased to about 2–3 tablespoons at each meal in the six month. Babies vary as much as adults in their appetite, so more precise quantities are hard to give. Give extra sucking time after spoon feeding to ensure baby is relaxed when he is put down after his feed.

After six months most babies will indicate how much food they are happy to take. Making sure he has had just sufficient and is contented, is quite different from giving him as much as he can be persuaded to eat to leave him bloated and immobile. The habit of always eating as much as you can possibly manage is learned young, and is a habit carried – dangerously – through life.

Foods to choose

There are four guidelines when giving food to your baby in the early months (or year) of feeding. These are listed below, and foods which you should *avoid* – or at least choose with great care – are listed in the chart opposite.

1. Food should be sufficiently easy for your baby to digest properly, and this will change according to his age. Some foods which are unsuitable at four to six months he should find easy to digest at seven to nine months, while others will still severely tax his digestive system until about two years. Individuals will vary in childhood as much as adulthood in what they can and cannot digest with ease, so that charts of suitable foods should be only taken as a guide.

2. Foods should be those currently believed to be the least likely to set up allergic reactions. Because there are now such large numbers of people showing varied allergies, a more careful choice of foods before six to seven months is vital. Those with a family history of allergies can presume their children could inherit a tendency and should take special care (see Chapter Nine).

3. Foods should be of a suitable nutritional value for your baby's present needs. Those foods which contain only calories and contribute little else, if anything, should be avoided or severely restricted. The baby's needs when mixed feeding starts are for those foods rich in vitamins and minerals that are insufficiently supplied by milk, as well as a little fibre, and protein.

Commercially prepared baby rice has vitamins and minerals added, and is a most useful part of a baby's diet under six to seven months as it is the one cereal that does not contain gluten. After this age, rice should be dropped largely in favour of a much wider range of cereals which will add to the diet.

4. Foods should be those which carry least risk of contamination by chemicals and sprays etc., or heavy metals such as lead. Some foods are more likely to be contaminated by germs in handling or contaminated in bad storage.

Food textures

Purées will need to be fairly runny at first; add sufficient boiled water, milk, fruit juice or unsalted vegetable water to gain this texture. A little fibrous material like skins of peas and corn do not appear to upset infants, but you can strain these out with a sieve or mouli the first few times they're given. Bran from grains is considered unsuitable until about six months; it tends to encourage the food to pass too quickly through the gut for good absorption to take place. Similarly the skins of most fruits are usually removed before cooking or puréeing, there being adequate fibre in the puréed flesh.

Foods which are too soft for easy feeding or because of their strong flavour need diluting (liver, for instance), can be combined with a firm purée of fruit or vegetables, or can have a little dehydrated baby rice sprinkled in to gain the ideal texture.

As soon as your baby manages to cope with sloppy foods in his mouth, begin to increase the density so that he acquires the skill of coping with thickened purées. These will remain comparatively smooth-textured in his first six months.

Finger foods

Small babies enjoy putting anything in their mouths; while you feed them they may try to grasp your spoon. While teething especially, firm items of food to gnaw may be a comfort.

Never leave a baby unaccompanied holding food in case he gags or chokes, which could be dangerous.

Suitable foods are: peeled, quartered and cored apple; peeled raw carrots, swede and parsnip; rusks; fingers of bread baked until crisp.

These foods will be sucked and gnawed but not truly eaten – firm items that do not break up in the mouth are best at this stage. Crisp vegetables will also help to clean the first tiny teeth. Avoid sweetened rusks and biscuits which will damage the teeth.

New foods

It is usual to give very simple purées of single foods at first – apple purée, carrot purée or rice cereal – before combining them with other purées or ingredients. The new food given is tried several times over a period of a few days before any other new food is added to the diet. This way it is possible to isolate with comparative ease any food upsetting your baby.

There is no need to use commercial baby products at this time although the specially reinforced baby rice is useful. The dessert commercial baby foods are a particularly poor choice since it is just as labour-saving and cost-effective – and considerably better for your baby – to have fresh fruit. Many foods you prepare for the family will be suitable for your baby, although jars or packets can be a useful standby.

CEREALS

Rice is the best choice of cereal at first. It is not as high in protein as are some others, but the protein in the high-protein cereals may contribute to allergies and should therefore be left until six to seven months (so do not select wheat, oats, mixed cereals, cereals with egg, muesli, wheatgerm and those marked as left to indicate gluten content). Whole-grain cereals are not usually given until five to six months.

Rice: Home-cooking your own rice for cereal is possible but is not the best choice since the commercial pre-cooked dry baby rice is much more convenient. Although refined it is enriched with high levels of iron, nicotinic acid, riboflavin and thiamin so will be of superior nutritional value. Buy the brand with the highest iron content and enriched with B vitamins, from your chemist or supermarket, and prepare it according to the manufacturer's instructions with six parts liquid to one part cereal at first.

VEGETABLES

These provide Vitamins A, C, E and K as well as valuable minerals. Different vegetables have different food values, and variety is an advantage. Give carrot first as it is the easiest to digest, then try combining it with other vegetables. Herbs and garlic may be used; herbs aid digestion.

Carrots: Prepare by washing, peeling and slicing. Cook in a very little *unsalted* water to half cover, then purée with all the cooking liquid for maximum food value. Alternatively, purée some carrot cooked with the family vegetables, so long as salt was omitted. Make to a soft purée with sufficient cooking liquid.

Next try some of the following.

Courgettes, green beans: Wash, cook and purée.

Parsnips, swede: Peel, cook and purée.

Celery, fennel, tomato: Wash, cook, purée and sieve.

Pumpkin, peas, sweetcorn: Cook and strain. Choose pale yellow corn if fresh, or frozen (never use tinned).

Follow with small quantities of other vegetables, combined with carrot or a more easily digested vegetable, as some of the following may cause wind.

Cauliflower, broccoli: High in food value, less likely to cause wind than many other greens; do not over-cook.

Sprouts, green cabbage: Boil but do not over-cook, or they will be more indigestible; combine with root vegetable purée.

Red/white cabbage: Boil quickly or casserole slowly, then purée.

Jerusalem artichokes: Scrape, boil and sieve.

Spinach: Cook in almost no water, and avoid early pickings of beet spinach which is high in oxalic acid. Mid-summer is better for spinach. Purée before or after cooking.

Onions, leeks: Serve only very small quantities.

Raw tomato: Dip in boiling water for 8 seconds then skin, quarter and cut out woody core. Pulp remainder.

FRUIT

Most fruit provides Vitamin C and minerals, and the yellow fruits contain Vitamin A. Apples or pears are a good first fruit; cooking or eating varieties can be used according to season. In early autumn, cookers may be very sour and as sugar should not be added, a less sharp eating apple may be preferred.

Apples, pears: Wash, peel, core and slice. Cook in a very little water, then purée with cooking liquid. Alternatively a little unsweetened apple from under a home-made pie or crumble can be puréed for baby. If you wish to add cereal to fruit you can mix in a little enriched baby rice. Very ripe pears may be puréed raw.

Try next some of the following.

Apples, raw: Very finely grate ripe apple – Cox type for preference.

Apricots: Stew in a little water, lift out skins and stones before puréeing. Tinned in own juice or water are suitable.

Bananas, raw: Choose ripe fruit with deep yellow skins, speckled brown, or firm brown skinned fruit that is not bruised. Mash with fork. Add a little boiled water if too sticky to swallow easily.

Cherries: Cooked and strained.

Citrus fruits: Orange, tangerine, grapefruit. Wash fruit, halve and squeeze out juice or peel. Purée with more pulpy fruit or vegetable – apple, banana, carrot. Wash baby's face after, as acid may cause a rash.

Peach, nectarine: Peel, stone and purée, give cooked or raw.

Pineapple: Cooked and puréed, fresh or tinned in own juice. Unsweetened pineapple juice can be combined with apple, banana or cereals.

Plums: Cooked or ripe raw, with peel removed. Give small quantity, as they may be laxative.

Exotic fruits: Kiwi, mango, paw-paw (papaya), peeled and cooked. Wash well, peel and purée ripe raw fruit and strain to remove seeds.

Dried fruit: Peaches, prunes, apricots, apples and pears – pour on boiling water (1½ cups to 1 cup fruit). Leave to soak overnight and stew until soft; purée finely. These tend to be laxative so do not give too much.

ANIMAL PROTEINS

Meat requiring a fairly long cooking time – all except liver and kidney – may not be practical to cook in small quantities for baby. So plan to cook as casseroles for all the family (without salt), or cook sufficient for several baby meals and freeze surplus.

Eggs: Try egg yolk only first – a teaspoon from a boiled egg. Later a little sieved hard-boiled egg. If tolerated well, try scrambled eggs, egg custards etc, but not if allergies run in the family.

Poultry: Well cooked chicken or turkey. Choose breast or thick thigh without skin. Chop first, and then purée adding vegetables.

Beef, veal and lamb: From well cooked lean roast meat, cooked without salt. Purée with vegetables and unseasoned vegetable water or boiled water.
From stews and casseroles prepared with minimum fat, no salt. Cook with vegetables, purée baby's portion before seasoning for family.
From grills, dice and purée with vegetables and boiled water.

Liver: Do not over-cook – simmer gently or steam with vegetables. Very easy to make to a fine purée, and is rich source of minerals and vitamins.

Kidney: Do not over-cook. Purée with vegetables.

Rabbit: Farmed, not wild game rabbit. Cook in casserole or stew with vegetables, then purée.

Six to eight months

Many basic foods will now have been tried and your baby may have had some food from family meals. He will soon be able to sit in a high chair and will start wanting to feed himself.

Cover the floor under the high chair with a plastic sheet so you will be more relaxed about his antics at meal-times. Use a plastic bucket bib when your baby is sitting well. He may also need an overall bib underneath with elasticated cuffs to keep him clean. Ensure you have a steady unbreakable bowl; a suction cup underneath is an asset. Also a tiny mug with small spout for drinking to keep spills to a minimum. Give baby his own spoon or finger foods if he keeps trying to grasp the one you are using. Let him play with spoon and finger food after meals if he is interested in increasing his skill.

By nine months a baby should be eating many of his meals at family meal-times, so gradually let him have his meals with you all whenever possible. Avoid hurried breakfast times and when you are trying to serve a more formal Sunday lunch. Choose those meals that are simple to serve and feed baby as well, to avoid a rushed and chaotic meal that no one will enjoy.

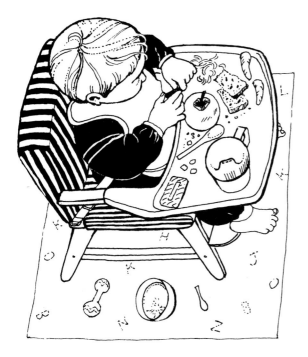

Food textures

Foods may be puréed less finely as baby acquires skill in dealing with food in his mouth; some items may be added mashed or diced, so long as most of the food is of a more puréed texture. The move from puréed to diced food is very slow and it is better to add only 1 teaspoon of coarse foods to half a cup of puréed food to gain a texture that will be acceptable to your baby. Gradually increase the amount of diced foods, ensuring that foods chosen for dicing are soft to chew – potato, carrot, peas – not firm meat that a baby will not be able to chew efficiently without plenty of teeth. The gums alone are quite sufficient for softer foods.

Finger foods

These become more important as more teeth are cut, and baby is more skilled with his hands. Never leave unattended with finger foods.

Suitable foods are: rusks and fingers of toasted wholemeal crust; peeled carrots, swede, parsnip, celery, cucumber; peeled pieces of firm apple.

You can also give him many foods being served at family meals – pieces of green beans, sprouts, cooked carrots, cauliflower and other cooked vegetables, fresh or raw fruit.

He may enjoy sucking a large smooth cooked chop or chicken bone if you have one handy.

New foods

Now he can afford to be a little more adventurous. Purée baby's food while dishing and seasoning the family meal. Leave to cool while you get the food and family to the table.

CEREALS
Choose a wide variety of high-protein cereals including whole grains, wheat, oats, barley, rye, wheatgerm, oat germ. These will be tolerated well by most babies without great risk of allergic reaction. Consult your doctor if baby develops prolonged tummy upsets with the introduction of wheat products (it may be coeliac disease, see Chapter Nine). Buy baby brands with the highest reinforcements of iron and B vitamins, and prepare according to manufacturer's instructions.

Home-made porridge: Serve this occasionally if you wish. Cook slowly after combining oats with cold milk, water or a mixture of the two for a creamy texture.

Muesli: After seven months you can choose baby muesli, but not the adult version (which has added sugar and a coarser texture). Add extra wheatgerm to any cereal, but allow to soak in milk to soften well before giving to baby. Combine with fruit if you wish (see the following pages for some ideas).

Whole-grain brown rice: This is best; add to casseroles or cook in covered container in water, until rice is soft and water absorbed. This will take about 40 minutes so prepare in bulk to freeze or serve to the family too. Do not rinse after cooking, or valuable B vitamins will be lost. Avoid polished white rice and rice starch; use rice cereals only rarely now – they do not contribute enough to the diet of the older baby.

Wholemeal flour, bread, pasta Choose these as often as possible; they are more nutritious than white. Avoid very coarse-grained brown bread, the types containing or topped with cracked wheat, which will be difficult to digest. 81% extraction brown flour is useful, better for sauces and suitable for most recipes calling for white flour. Avoid cornflour and commercial goods with modified food starch. Main dishes may have brown bread or wholemeal pasta added to the purées. Add a small piece of bread or a little cooked pasta when puréeing vegetables with cheese or meat. Brown, white and green pastas are available in all shapes and sizes, and all are suitable for baby (although brown, because of the extra goodness, is preferable).

Fingers of toasted crust of bread instead of commercial sweetened rusks will keep him happily entertained while you finish preparing his food. Cook in oven, under grill, or in toaster.

VEGETABLES

He can try many more now, including the protein-rich pulses. Parsley or watercress chopped over other vegetables not only do baby good, but make the food look more attractive.

Green vegetables, cauliflower: Increase the quantity of these as soon as they can be eaten without causing indigestion. Try not to waste the cooking liquid but use in purée, or even as a drink.

Potatoes: Choose those without any traces of green, and give old in preference to new. Boil or bake in their skins. Do not keep cooking water – discard this in favour of other vegetable water. Use food mill or masher – not blender – to purée, otherwise they become sticky or waxy.

Beetroots: They can be given to baby raw. You can also foil-wrap and bake whole beetroot in the oven for one to two hours until the skin will rub off; alternatively steam or boil. Do not be alarmed; red beetroot staining may pass through to baby's nappy.

Pulses: At seven months try giving cooked orange or red lentils which are quick to cook and need no soaking. Other pulses or legumes need soaking before cooking well. All are suitable at seven to eight months: split yellow, green and black-eyed peas; grey, green, brown and red lentils; butter, kidney and flageolet beans. Soya beans are a particularly useful substitute for meat as they are complete protein, while other peas and beans are only incomplete proteins. For ease, cook beans etc. in large quantities (without salt) and freeze. Avoid tinned beans as all contain salt, but you can give them after eight months.

Yams, sweet potatoes: Buy good sound yams only. Cook in peel, steaming for 30 minutes or baking for 1 hour. Scoop flesh out of skin, put in food mixer or use masher (not a blender).

Leek, onion: Only small quantities, cooked, until after eight months.

Parsley, watercress: Purée finely, cooked or raw. Very good nutritional value.

Avocado: Mash ripe avocado, adding milk or lemon juice to soften.

FRUIT

Give ripe fresh fruits in season for variety, goodness – and pleasure! Babies enjoy lots of different flavours and textures at this stage.

Currants, gooseberries: Stew and strain off seeds, combine with apples or pears at first to make a firmer, milder purée.

Citrus fruit: Give segments of orange or grapefruit, satsuma etc., finely chopped or puréed.

Cherries: Purée with skins, and remove stones.

Apricots, peaches, nectarines: Purée raw if ripe.

Melon: Purée raw. Avoid watermelon which carries a slight risk of contamination.

Pineapple: Purée raw in blender.

ANIMAL PROTEINS

Dishes should still be unseasoned, but many more tastes will be acceptable now.

Eggs: Whole egg will be tolerated by most infants now. Those with eczema or other allergies who may not tolerate it should wait until up to two years. Give scrambled, boiled or omelettes with vegetables, or use in custards and desserts.

Poultry, rabbit: From unseasoned family dishes or cooked for baby – do not give fried, or with spices, only herbs.

Beef, veal, lamb: From unseasoned family dishes omitting pastry. Give only lean meat free of gristle – no fried foods, sausages, bought pies etc.

Liver, offal: From slow-cooked family casseroles, or cooked lightly for baby. Give once a week.

Cheese: Cheddar type, cottage and curd cheese. Do not cook if possible. Stir into hot purées to melt. Cottage and curd cheese may be puréed with cold fruit or vegetables.

Yogurt: Plain yogurt may be given as is, or with home-made fruit purées. Avoid commercial fruit yogurts.

White fish: Fine-textured sole, plaice, whiting or small fillets of haddock. Cook gently in milk or steam on a plate over a pan of vegetables, or cover and bake in oven or microwave. Do not over-cook or fibres will toughen. Avoid smoked or oily fish and shellfish. Avoid bones by *very* careful checking.

Eight to fifteen months

By this stage, your baby will be quite ready to join family meals. These meal-times should be pleasant, social occasions – they are not the time to discuss finances, politics, discipline or any similar subject that will lead to tension. Infants and young children are quick to sense this and create a diverting scene. Throwing tantrums and food, refusing to eat generally, set the pattern of unhappy meal-times with all resorting to TV meals, eating they know not what most of the time.

Not all family meals will be suitable for baby; the times may be wrong and food inappropriate. As far as possible you should try to ensure that meals are partly or largely suitable for your baby. He should not be eating different food at a majority of meals.

Now that he is joining the rest of the family regularly, be aware that babies and toddlers can be very sensitive to the attitude of other members of the family to food. A faddy Daddy, brothers or sisters who will not eat green vegetables or salad, complain about meat being fatty, and who consistently list their likes and dislikes at meal-times, will need to be retrained well before your infant reaches the family table. To save later tantrums, your patience – and the ultimate health of your baby – lay down a few rules for yourself and the rest of the family:

1. Remove as much fat from meat as possible. It is very bad for all of you.

2. Green vegetables should be eaten for good health. If any members of the family will not eat them, always cook and serve a variety of vegetables – peas, carrots, cauliflower – and allow all to help themselves to what they *do* enjoy. Pushing the unpopular is usually counter-productive. Set a good example by serving carefully cooked greens regularly and enjoy them yourself.

3. Do not allow any member of the family to say 'I don't like . . .' Only allow 'I prefer . . .' or 'I do like . . .' If you are going to give soft margarine instead of butter, for instance, explain *why*.

4. Keep a firm regime about between-meal snacks if your family are prone to being faddy. There is nothing like hunger to make them enjoy sensible, well cooked food. If they are not hungry at meal-times they are much more likely to be picky. If your family need biscuits at elevenses and tea give them, but if lunch and high tea or supper is not eaten afterwards then keep the biscuit tin empty.

5. Expect people to have preferences in food; a few reasonable dislikes should be accepted. Normally in families the preferences are inherited – being squeamish about some offal, not liking eggs (this is often a true allergy), disliking broad beans (they give some people severe wind). As a result these foods are normally not met with at home, and only encountered when eating out. Respect a few preferences and you are more likely to have cooperation overall.

Food textures

It is very tempting at this stage, for speed and ease and to avoid messy clearing up at the end of a meal, to keep shovelling food into your baby and get the whole job of feeding over as soon as possible. It is tempting too to keep the food soft and pappy so that it can be quickly swallowed down spoon by spoon while you are busy with other members of the family.

Continuing to give food in this consistently soft, pappy and bland state will make him very late in developing the art of chewing. It will make him very lazy and reluctant to chew if eating is made too easy for too long. Chewing stimulates the flow of blood in the jaws; this helps good growth of jaws, so allowing more room for teeth. It will also help keep the gums and small new teeth in good condition.

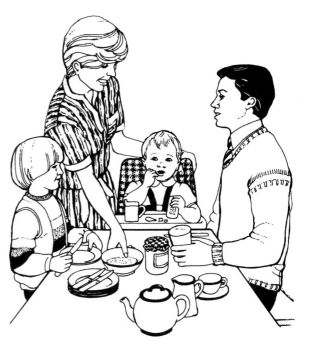

Meal-Time Safety

● Choose a free-standing high-chair with care. Tall chairs to put at the dining table are not safe, as they are easily toppled over if baby pushes against the table.

● Choose a good safety harness to secure child in chair and always use even if you think you are going to remain in the room. You may be called away in an emergency, or to the phone or door. You don't want to return to find your baby on the floor.

● Choose suitable protective clothing for baby, and covering for the floor.

● Do not use cloth on the table. Baby may pull scalding food onto himself.

● Do not place hot food or drink within a baby or toddler's arms' reach in case he grasps it and tries to feed himself.

At six to eight months diced or coarser food was introduced. This proportion can now be stepped up, with the inclusion of less soft diced foods. Chewing raw carrots and apples particularly stimulates the flow of saliva to rinse the mouth of food particles, and the friction will also clean any build-up of sweet or cereal matter which is so damaging to the teeth.

Finger foods

During this period a baby will learn to feed himself quite efficiently if given the opportunity. From eight months he will become increasingly adept at putting food in his mouth, albeit with his fingers at first. He will attempt to pick up thick purées and any diced foods – peas, carrots, corn, beans, diced potatoes, fish, cheese, eggs – to help feed himself. He will enjoy picking up pasta, rice, bread and fruits. Do not mix foods up if this is not how he likes them – he may prefer to have small piles of pasta; diced or grated cheese; diced chicken or other meats; diced or small, whole cooked vegetables and a few larger pieces of salad items.

What he may *also* enjoy is dropping his food on the floor. Do not let this become a game. Always presume that when a baby drops food he is no longer hungry; remove it and he will quickly get the message.

Avoid small pieces of hard food which might easily cause choking. Keep raw vegetables in long sticks for chewing.

As soon as baby is skilled with his fingers let him try to use a spoon and fingers, or spoon and fork, but do not force this. He will become frustrated and bad-tempered if hungry, and foods keep rolling off the spoon because of his ineptitude. A dish of finger foods for him to start on will give you a few moment's peace to serve the rest of the family. You can then give the wetter foods with two spoons, one for you to use and one for him to have a go. If he prefers to use his fingers for sticky purées, do not discourage him at such a young age. He will probably be sucking enough food off his fingers, and this is not the age to worry about social refinements. So long as floor and baby are well protected from mess and no brothers and sisters are within sticky arms' reach, being independent in his feeding is of great value. It not only frees the mother to eat her own meals and look after the whole family, but it also prevents the battle of wills that so easily develops when a baby comes to realize that he can make his mother cross by refusing to eat food or by keeping her waiting. He needs to accept that he puts food into his own mouth as and when he needs it, and that eating is not a game nor a battle of wits.

New foods

If you wish your child to only eat brown bread, wholesome breakfast cereal, and no sugar, pop, junk food etc., you must start this practice while they are very young. Once they reach fifteen months many children have become very set in their ideas. Once they have tasted Frosties it will be a constant battle to re-wean them through their early years away from such highly sweetened cereal.

CEREALS

Do not give sugar-, chocolate- or honey-coated cereals as finger foods; they are bad for the teeth – and for the future. What they have never tasted they will not clamour for. There are plenty of excellent breakfast cereals reinforced with minerals and vitamins with a high fibre content and a minimum of sweetening. The best include ProNutro, Weetabix, Shredded Wheat, Wheat Flakes and the chain-store varieties, Readybrek, porridge oats and porridge with bran. Some brands of muesli and granola are very heavily sweetened which is a pity; health-food shops stock less sweet alternatives. Rice and corn cereals are low in bran and often protein, so are not the best choice unless eaten with extra bran or All-bran.

Breakfast cereals are *not sour*, so they do not need any sugar sprinkled on top. This is an unnecessarily bad habit. Sprinkle on wheatgerm, ground nuts or chopped dried fruit for a varied topping.

Pasta: Use wholemeal, or pasta enriched with egg.

Bread: Rusks or biscuits. Choose either crisp foods which can be gnawed and sucked, or very soft food moistened with milk so it can be easily swallowed. Fruit loaves are best soaked in milk or toasted until dry. White bread will be too chewy for many infants, but more crumbly wholemeal may be easier and can be spread sparingly with curd cheese, soft margarine, butter, honey, Marmite, malt extract or smooth jams or jellies.

VEGETABLES

There are now few vegetables a baby may not eat. Since salt is now permissible a wide range of tinned vegetables can be used. The wider the range given at eight months the better accustomed baby will become to variety, and you will avoid fussiness and refusals later.

Baked beans: Very popular with children and adults, they are very cheap and very nutritious. Be happy to use regularly as a near-perfect convenience food. Brands vary – choose those with fewest additions and most beans per can; not the cheapest. They do contain sugar and modified starch, but their nutritional advantages far outweigh these.

Butter, kidney, other tinned beans, sweetcorn: Do not purée with salted liquid from can, but this may be added to casseroles, mince, stews etc. for stock if no other salt or salted stock cube is used. Very convenient to avoid long cooking.

Mushrooms: Use only farmed mushrooms, not wild, which can cause food poisoning. Give only a trace of mushroom the first time – a little sauce from a meat casserole with mushrooms, for instance. If this is tolerated increase the quantity next time and then give freely. Avoid until at least two years in families with a history of mushroom allergy.

Aubergine, peppers: Give cooked in casseroles, ratatouille, etc.

Onions, leeks: Large quantities can usually be tolerated well. Cut leek across in fine strips and cook quickly in a few tablespoons of stock or water; excellent in soups or combined with other vegetables.

Salads: Puréed or very finely chopped raw spinach, watercress or lettuce can be given. Also finely grated celery, cucumber, fennel, carrot. You could also serve some cooked ingredients: these can be moistened with a little mayonnaise (not salad cream), yogurt, cottage, curd or cream cheese combined with milk, peanut butter mixed with hot milk, or with purées of lentils, soya beans or other vegetables.

Peanuts: Very finely grind to make paste, or choose smooth peanut butter with few additives from your health-food shop. Mix to a soft not tacky texture with milk, water, fruit juice or vegetable purée, otherwise it will just stick to baby's mouth and make him gag.

FRUIT

Many different fruit can now be given, cooked or raw, whole or in chunks as finger foods. Baby's tastes should be widening weekly!

Berries: Raspberries, blackberries, bilberries, loganberries can be cooked or raw, puréed and sieved at first, then try a little with seeds which is tolerated well by most babies at this stage. Whole fruit can be given at over one year.

Strawberries: These can cause a rash in many, so give only a little at first. If tolerated well, mash finely or purée.

Grapes: Seeded or seedless. Chop firm sweet grapes with skins on. Do not give whole until at least one year, or when chewing is efficient, to prevent choking.

Currants, goose-berries:	Seeds may be gradually tolerated in cooked fruit.	**Pork, ham:**	Pork is a difficult meat to digest. It should be very lean and very well cooked if given to a child, especially under two years. Pork carries some small risk from a parasite which is why it should always be very well cooked. Ham, cold and sliced, can be bought from a reliable clean shop. It is better to buy from shops that have a special cold meat or meat and cheese counter where tongs are used and where money is not handled.
Citrus fruits:	Try segments roughly chopped after eight months, and whole after one year or when baby chews well.		
Apples, pears, peaches, nectarines:	Coarsely grate, mash or give in fingers raw.		
Cherries:	Serve whole only after one year, with stones removed until three years old.		
Melon:	All but watermelon, mashed or in fingers.	**Milk:**	1¼–1¾ pints (700 ml–1 litre) should be taken daily at eight months, but will probably decrease to less than 1 pint (575 ml) at ten months. Doorstep cow's milk or full cream UHT milk can be used. Avoid skimmed or dried milk designed for adult consumption.
Pineapple:	Finely chopped or puréed. Chunks may be given as finger food.		
Rhubarb:	Give only occasionally. Always serve cooked, removing all trace of leaves. Sweeten with honey or brown sugar.		

ANIMAL PROTEINS
Keep fat to a minimum in the diet. This means a very little pastry in meat pies etc.

Yogurt:	Can be counted as part of the milk intake. Avoid as long as possible the commercial fruit yogurt; although convenient they contain little fruit, a lot of sugar (*about 1 tablespoon*), as well as artificial colouring and flavouring, etc.	**Fish:**	A wide range of white fish can be given once or twice a week at least. The coarser textured white fish and trout are suitable, whether fresh or frozen. Oily fish – mackerel, herring, and tinned sardines etc. – are not very suitable until after fifteen months.
		Beef, lamb, poultry:	Meat that is home-cooked, quickly cooled and stored in the fridge up to three days may be given to baby cold, or added to vegetable purées or vegetables with sauces or gravy.

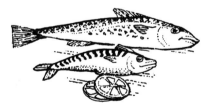

Equipment for preparing baby foods

You don't need *special* equipment for preparing baby foods – most households already possess most of the following list – but it's appropriate to know what can be most useful. In many cases, all that will be needed is a good mashing fork!

But the principal thing to remember is hygiene. There is no point in sterilising bottles and spoons and dishes impeccably until solid foods are established, and then letting standards drop. Complete hygiene is still vital.

Rinse all baby utensils in boiling water. Well wash separately from family utensils before use. Plastic utensils such as spoons and spatulas, can be kept in bottle sterilising solution. Do not wipe dry on a tea towel, which may carry germs, but dry on kitchen paper, or use wet. Items taken straight from a dishwasher are sterile. These precautions are necessary in the first seven months, after which normal to very good household standards will be adequate. It is presumed that food will not be in contact with these utensils for very long, which minimises the risk of contamination, *not* as in the case of feeding bottles, which must be more carefully sterilised. When any member of the family has infections, like a cold, greater care is needed to prevent the spread of germs. Wash all baby's utensils and store separately unless a dish-washer is used.

Puréeing equipment

Purées will be the first solid food prepared, and the following are what I have found most useful. Always rinse utensils with boiling water before use if possible.

Nylon sieves are good for small quantities and for fruit and tomatoes. Especially suitable when wishing to separate seeds from berries and currants for small babies. They are not good for meat, fish or green vegetables which will not rub through well.

Metal sieves are good for small quantities of carrots, cauliflower, potatoes and other root vegetables. Green vegetables have to be somewhat overcooked to go through well so do not use for these. Good for kidney, liver and fine fleshed fish (plaice), but more difficult for other meat and fish, and not at all good for acid fruits which gain a metallic flavour.

Purée DOs and DON'Ts

DO   add hot soapy water to processors and blenders, and switch on to thoroughly clean. Rinse under tap. Do not immerse or machine wash unless recommended.

DO   chop meat and firm food in dice before puréeing. It will be easier for your. machine.

DO   add liquid first to electric blenders. Food will turn more easily if wet. Add solid items to purée gradually.

DON'T   use coffee mills unless they can be adequately cleaned.

DON'T   use blenders designed for milk shakes. They are not strong enough for puréeing foods.

A **potato masher** is ideal for cooked fruit, banana, ripe pears, avocado and cooked root vegetables, kidney and liver, particularly from nine months when lumpier food is eaten.

A stainless steel **grater** is useful with star-shaped grater surface to grate fruits to a pulp, plus a scoop-shaped shredding surface. Most useful for firm cheese. Scrub clean with nailbrush when washing.

A **Mouli** and other hand-turned food blenders are useful for small quantities. Good for fruits, including those with seeds and pips, root vegetables, green vegetables, and for liver, chicken breast, kidney, fish, mince. Not very good for fibrous meat, stewing steak, roast meat.

Electric blenders are good for larger quantities for freezing or serving to whole family. There has to be sufficient to turn on the blade, so 1 cupful is more successful than 1 tablespoon. Will purée all foods. Good for wet fish, purées of fruit, soups, stews, but not suitable where seeds must be separated from currants and berries for small baby under twelve to fifteen months. It will be necessary to sieve food as well to separate seeds. They are not suitable for drier mixtures of meat and vegetables if these are required (the food does not turn easily on the blades), but most infants prefer to eat their food well moistened. Not always good with tougher meats and roast meats, which may remain fairly coarse. This will depend on machine.

Food processors are good with large quantities, and with tougher coarse-textured meat and vegetables which will become very fine. Not good with small quantities of moist food which will tend to be thrown up the sides and not come in contact with blade. Best with very wet or dry foods for efficient processing. Foods with pips and seeds may also need straining.

Hand-held liquidisers are cheap and useful for small quantities, and can be used in a cup or deep pan, but not good for tougher meat and more fibrous foods.

Cookers and cooking utensils

Again, you will already possess many of these but a few are more useful than others. Continue the same high standards of hygiene.

Coddlers (small pots with screw tops), small cups or jars covered with foil, or 'boil-in-the-bag' bags, are useful for steaming small quantities of food. The container can be placed in pan with fitting lid and ½–1 inch (1–2 cm) water, and a variety of goods can be cooked simultaneously: a pot of custard, bag of apples, cup of fish and peas. No special steamer is necessary and if food is cooked and cooled in covered container, some pots or bags may be used later in the day (see *One-Pot Cooking*).

A **small thick pan with tight-fitting lid** is a basic and essential piece of equipment, so useful for one-pot cooking. Only a small amount of liquid is used for this, so no valuable nutrients are thrown away. Food is added to the pan according to cooking time; meat first as it takes longest to cook, then root vegetables, lastly green or frozen vegetables or fish. Food can then be mashed with potato masher for toddler food, or puréed for baby. Sufficient is freshly cooked for just one baby's meal unless extra is prepared for mother (see *Lunch-time Recipes for Mother and Baby*).

Choose a stainless steel or enamel pan with a thick base, or food will burn easily. Do not choose an iron pan; again foods burn too easily. Choose a non-stick pan if you wish. If you choose an aluminium pan, do not scour the inside heavily or regularly with scouring pads, powders or creams. The shiny aluminium exposed is more susceptible to combining with food to create toxic aluminium salts, and babies, small children and expectant mothers are most at risk of exposure to this. Polish up the outside of the pans if you wish but not the inside.

The dull surface of aluminium, which is an oxide, is less likely to dissolve in foods but even this will be removed when exposed to acid fruits and vegetables. Avoid cooking the following in aluminium pans:

Tomatoes	Apples	Damsons
Spinach	Rhubarb	Pineapples
Vinegar	Citrus fruits	Strawberries
Pickles	Apricots	Gooseberries
Chutney	Plums	Currants
Yogurt	Grapes	Raspberries

The one-pot and coddling methods of cooking are particularly effective in **pressure cookers**, and vitamins and minerals will not be lost to any great extent. A variety of items may be cooked together in baskets, to come in contact with steam for slower cooking foods (potatoes and meat), or in lightly covered containers. There is a minimum of washing up using this method, and one session can prepare main dish for lunch, plus fruit purée for later use (quickly cover in its container, and store in fridge). Another useful aspect of pressure cooking: if you run out of bottle sterilising tablets or fluid, just bring bottles and teats up to full pressure to sterilise. Store in covered pan or make up feed and store in refrigerator.

An **electric slow cooker** is useful for making large quantities of meat and poultry very tender, and retains vitamins and minerals well. Always add *boiling* liquid to chicken casseroles so bacteria are killed quickly. Boil any dish containing kidney beans well before serving or adding to casserole (for at least 15 minutes) as slow-cooking does not reach a high enough temperature.

A **microwave oven** retains vitamins and minerals very well, and is very quick and easy. Just place items in covered Pyrex pot or bowl for those needing moist heat (green vegetables, meat and white fish); others may be placed on plate or dish. Particularly suitable for thawing frozen foods which can be safely and quickly boiled. Excellent for heating baby's bottle.

Baked foil packs are small packets of food or covered dishes which can be baked in the oven for baby's meal. Moisten lightly before covering. This is only cost-effective if the oven is used for family dishes or baking. Ideal temperature around 325°F/160°C/Gas 3, but this may depend on other use of the oven. Roasting temperatures are a bit hot and likely to dry food.

Freezing baby foods

Freezing is the newest food storage revolution, and frozen food – if frozen properly – retains most of its texture, flavour and nutritional properties. But hygiene – whether for family or baby – must be impeccable, and the basic freezing rules must be adhered to very carefully.

If you wish to freeze food, for the family in general, or for a baby, it should be done at below 0°F (−18°C). A basic requirement of any freezer is that it can freeze food to this temperature or below, within twenty-four hours. Only appliances with *four* stars (one big star and three smaller ones) are for *freezing* foods: all other freezer sections attached to fridges are for *storage of frozen foods* only (one star keeps already frozen food for one week; two stars will keep frozen food for up to a month; three stars will keep frozen food for up to three months).

Packaging must be sterile – use special freezing films, polythene bags, foil or rigid boxes – and the food must be cold before freezing commences (otherwise the residual heat will affect the temperature in the freezer and thus other frozen foods).

Quantities to freeze

First foods will only be consumed 1 teaspoon to 1 tablespoon at a time. Purée finely and freeze in ice cubes until just frozen, knock out then store in airtight bags.

Second-stage foods will be needed in quantities of about 1–4 tablespoons. These will not need to be puréed quite so finely. Freeze in clean small yogurt pots, or place large spoonfuls in dollops on clean baking tray. Open-freeze until hard (a few hours) then knock off and store in airtight bags. One, two or three will make a meal, according to baby's age, and another advantage is that they thaw fairly swiftly.

Third-stage food will be taken 3 tablespoons to ½ cup or more as appetite increases. Food should be slightly lumpy. Freeze in strong freezer bags or containers.

Thawing

Thaw small quantities of food designed for baby at room temperature for half an hour or more quickly in microwave, normal oven or, if in suitable container, in pan of boiling water. Bring food to boil, then cool quickly. Serve immediately.

Alternatively, food may be thawed in fridge over-night and served cold. Suitable for fruit purées, home-made mousses and fruit crumbles.

Thaw large items for family use in fridge for twelve to twenty-four hours (cooked casseroles, soups, stews and raw chicken meat). Always bring to boil, do not just warm. Cook frozen fish, fruit and vegetables from frozen as far as possible for maximum food value.

When using frozen fruit purées for making mousses and ice creams, thaw covered in fridge or at room temperature. Make dessert and return to freezer. Acid fruits are safe to thaw and to re-freeze without boiling – for strawberry ice cream or raspberry mousses. Freeze these in larger containers and the required amount for a serving can be spooned out, frozen. Fill space with crumpled greaseproof paper or foil to prevent excessive ice build-up.

Safe Freezing

DO read a good freezer book for the best advice before freezing foods for a baby.

DO store and freeze food in coldest part of freezer (often near the walls), and turn freezer to lowest temperature beforehand.

DO pack food in suitable quantities to avoid wastage (see below).

DON'T re-freeze food which has thawed, but defrosted *raw* food may be cooked and then frozen again for later use.

DO chill cooked food quickly and freeze as soon as cold.

DO purée leftovers from freshly cooked meal immediately after meal and freeze. Do not freeze foods, especially vegetables, that have been kept hot and will have lost food value.

DO wrap food carefully to avoid loss of moisture and food value. Freezer 'burn' does no harm nutritionally, but it spoils the texture and quality.

DO use frozen baby foods within one month.

Buying and storing baby foods

Meat

DO thaw frozen meat before cooking, especially poultry: twenty-four hours at room temperature for chicken, three days for turkey approximately. There is *high* risk of food poisoning for all if not properly thawed and *well* cooked. Never stuff centre cavity of birds as this increases risk of food poisoning (stuffing can be cooked in separate small pan).

DON'T buy cooked meats for a baby. You never know what contamination they have encountered.

DO use all meat as quickly as possible. After purchase store in fridge or freezer.

DO buy only very lean mince from a very reputable source. Most mince is too fatty and unsuitable for baby under about nine months. Brown mince first before adding anything else, and strain off all melted fat.

DON'T handle raw meat, especially chicken, then touch cooked meats or food – you may pass on dangerous bacteria.

DO wash all chopping boards thoroughly after preparing meat and poultry.

Fish

DO use only freshest fish – there should be no smell of ammonia, especially on oily fish like mackerel. If in doubt choose frozen.

DON'T give baby shellfish, mussels, prawns, etc.

DO wash fresh fish well in cold running water.

DON'T thaw fish slowly. Cook from frozen whenever possible. Frozen fish is often of better quality than so-called fresh wet fish (which may have been already frozen and thawed, and certainly will have taken some time to get to the shop from the sea or river).

DO store fresh fish in fridge and use same day.

Eggs

DO store dome up without washing for maximum shelf life.

DO store in fridge or cool larder.

Milk

DON'T leave on doorstep, for sun spoils food value.

DO store in *bottle* in fridge.

DON'T pour into jug, except for immediate use at table. There is greater risk of contamination.

DO store away from strong-smelling foods: fish and strong cheese can taint the flavour, although it is safe to drink.

DO treat UHT milk like ordinary milk once open.

Cheese

DO wrap loosely and then store in box to prevent formation of mould (on cheese this is not a health risk) or tainting flavour of other foods.

DO freeze what you will not use immediately.

Green Vegetables

DO keep in polythene bag in refrigerator.

DO wash thoroughly before cooking – they may have been contaminated with sprays.

DON'T cook in a lot of water and throw the dissolved minerals and vitamins away.

DON'T overcook – they become *less digestible* and considerably less in food value.

DON'T buy more than you will use in two to three days – they will be losing Vitamin C.

DON'T wash, slice or soak long before cooking.

DON'T cut vegetables too much before cooking in water or most food value will be lost.

DO cook green vegetables *as fast* as possible until barely tender.

DO have lid only half on when cooking green vegetables. Tightly covering causes an unappetising musty smell, enough to put children off greens for life.

DON'T keep vegetables hot – cook and serve immediately for maximum food value.

If all vegetable cooking water is reserved for soup and sauces and only a moderate amount used dissolved minerals will not be lost.

Root Vegetables

DON'T keep potatoes, especially new potatoes, in daylight. They will become green, toxic and sprout more readily.

DO use new potatoes within one to three days of purchase. They will have more Vitamin C, less risk of turning green, and skins will remove more easily.

DON'T store onions in the dark, otherwise they will sprout and become soft.

DO keep all vegetables in a cool place. They store well with little loss of food value.

DO wash all vegetables well before cooking or peeling. They may be contaminated.

DON'T peel vegetables unless really necessary.

DO use a potato peeler if you must peel – potatoes, carrots etc. Most of the food value is just under the skin.

DO cook in a very little water in covered pan.

DO reserve all vegetable water for use in cooking.

DO add *dried milk* powder to mashed potato for baby, and to vegetable water for white sauces, carrots, cauliflower, etc.

DO bake vegetables in skins – potatoes, etc.

Fruit and Salads

DO wash well just before preparing to remove contamination from chemical sprays, etc., even if peeling.

DO buy only what you will use in one to four days, except citrus fruit, apples, unripe bananas and pears, which store quite well.

DO leave skins on apples, pears, cucumbers, which are perfectly edible for all but the smallest babies.

DO serve food raw whenever possible.

DO keep peel of oranges, lemons and satsumas, etc. (drop in freezer). They are excellent for flavouring and have food value.

DO give fruit whole or as unstrained juice. The membranes add much to the diet. Excellent though fruit juices are, the whole fruits are better nutritionally.

Tins, Jars and Packets

DO always note contents of convenience foods. They are listed in *descending* order of amount – the largest quantity first.

DON'T buy bulging and damaged tins.

DO choose foods with fewest additives, colourings, flavourings, preservatives, etc.

DO choose fruits tinned in own juices, without sugar, available in some supermarkets.

DO wash top of tins before opening.

DO check tins on opening. Food should be drawn in, not contents spilled out, if foods are correctly canned. Vacuum jars should make a 'pop' on unscrewing if correctly packed.

DO use liquid in cans of fruit (if unsweetened) and vegetables – about one-third of the minerals and vitamins may be dissolved in this. Juices or sweetened tinned fruits are *too sweet* for a baby and will encourage a craving for sugared food.

DON'T store food in opened cans. Turn into clean covered container.

DON'T spoon food out of jar into baby's mouth and return remainder to fridge for next day. Food will be contaminated by bacteria and enzymes from baby's mouth. Spoon what will be required with clean spoon into baby's dish and place remainder of jar straight in fridge for later use. (This method is not suitable for *tins* of baby food).

DO choose instant dried baby food in preference to tins or jars when you start mixed feeding with commercial products. Your baby may only want ½–2 teaspoons of the dried food which you can mix to a sloppy purée with warm, boiled water. Very small quantities can be tried and the packet of dry food resealed carefully for later use.

Storage Times of Opened Tins and Jars in Fridge

Fruit in juice or syrup	4–6 days
Evaporated milk	4 days
Tomato purée and sauces	4 days
Citrus and tomato juice	3 days
Meat, soup and vegetables	2 days
Fish, poultry and baby foods	1 day

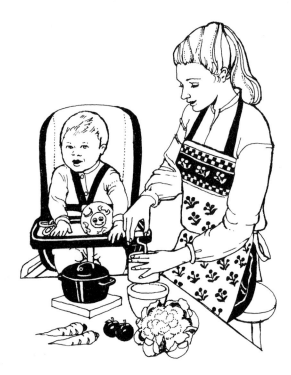

Baby and family meals

You will be more tempted to give baby home-cooked food if this is made as labour-saving as possible. Plan baby's meals to fit in with your own or family meals, or cook and freeze for greater convenience.

To save on time, washing up *and* gas or electricity, the first two sections are for recipes which can be made in one pan, whether in larger quantities for freezing for later use, or for two courses to be cooked simultaneously. With much the same idea in mind, I give some recipes which will feed baby, but at the same time – with a little adaptation – serve as a soup or toast-topper for mother's lunch. Salads are important for everyone, including baby, and there are guidelines for adapting family meals and puddings, and improving favourite recipes, so that they are suitable for *every* member of the family.

All recipes in the following sections are suitable from six to eight months on, and can be puréed or mashed according to baby or toddler's age. Extra water may need to be added: this will depend on how much is lost in evaporation and how moist your baby needs his food. If too runny, add a little baby rice cereal to thicken.

One-pot cooking

When small quantities of food are needed you will not want half a dozen pans on the cooker for a few spoons of food. The following recipes may be made in the small quantity specified, or larger quantity for freezing.

LIVER, CAULIFLOWER AND TOMATO

1 portion	*For freezing*
Small piece cauliflower	¼ whole cauliflower
½ teaspoon soft margarine	1 teaspoon soft margarine
1–2 oz (30–60 g) chicken or lamb's liver	½ lb (225 g) chicken or lamb's liver
1 teaspoon flour	1 tablespoon flour
3–4 tablespoons water	½ pint (300 ml) water
1 tomato	4 tomatoes

Cooking time: 15 minutes
Wash cauliflower and chop. Melt fat in pan, dust liver with flour and sauté gently 1–2 minutes on each side. Add water, cauliflower and washed halved tomatoes. Cover and cook 10–12 minutes until cauliflower is soft. Remove tomato skins before serving.

LAMB CHOP, POTATO AND CORN

1 portion	*For freezing*
1 small lamb chop	2–3 larger lamb chops
¼ pint (150 ml) water	½–¾ pint (300–425 ml) water
¼ potato	1 potato
1 very small bay leaf	2–3 small bay leaves
1–2 teaspoons sweetcorn, frozen	2–3 tablespoons sweetcorn, frozen
1 teaspoon chopped parsley	1 tablespoon chopped parsley

Cooking time: 30 minutes
Trim excess fat off chop, cook in water with bay leaf and well scrubbed potato for 20–25 minutes. Lift out and skin potato, add corn to pan, cook for 4–7 minutes. Discard bay leaf, cut meat off bone, return to pan with potato and parsley.

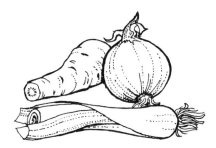

CHICKEN WITH BROWN RICE AND BROAD BEANS

1 portion	*For freezing*
1 small joint chicken	2 joints chicken
¼ pint (150 ml) water	½–¾ pint (300–425 ml) water
½–1 tablespoon brown rice	3 tablespoons brown rice
1 tablespoon broad beans (fresh or frozen)	3 tablespoons broad beans (fresh or frozen)
1–2 teaspoons lemon juice	1 tablespoon lemon juice

Cooking time: 40–45 minutes

Cook chicken in pan with water and brown rice. Simmer for 35 minutes then add beans. Cook for 5–10 minutes or until all are tender. If skins on beans are tough these should be removed. Discard skin and bone of chicken, return meat to pan with lemon juice.

KIDNEY, TOMATO AND PASTA

1 portion	*For freezing*
1 lamb's kidney	4 lamb's kidneys
1 teaspoon sunflower margarine	2 teaspoons sunflower margarine
¼ pint (150 ml) water	½ pint (300 ml) water
1 tablespoon pasta shapes	Small handful pasta shapes
1 tomato	4 tomatoes

Cooking time: 15–20 minutes

Halve kidney, snip out core with scissors and remove skin. Fry cut side up in hot fat until lightly brown, turn over and cook briefly. Add water, pasta and halved tomato; simmer until pasta is cooked. Remove tomato skin.

BACON WITH SPROUTS

1 portion	*For freezing*
1 rasher of lean bacon	4 rashers of lean bacon
4 tablespoons water	¼ pint (150 ml) water
2 Brussels sprouts	8 Brussels sprouts
4 tablespoons milk	¼ pint (150 ml) milk
1 teaspoon wholemeal flour	1 tablespoon wholemeal flour
1 teaspoon finely chopped parsley	1 tablespoon finely chopped parsley

Cooking time: 10–15 minutes

Fry chopped bacon until fat runs, add water, bring to boil and add quartered sprouts. Simmer until tender. Mix milk and flour to thin paste. Pour into pan, stir briskly and bring to the boil to thicken, then add parsley.

WHITE FISH AND GREEN BEANS

1 portion	*For freezing*
2 oz (60 g) coley or plaice	½ lb (225 g) coley or plaice
⅛–¼ pint (75–150 ml) milk	½ pint (300 ml) milk
1 tablespoon fresh or frozen green beans	½ lb (225 g) fresh or frozen green beans
1 teaspoon soft margarine	3 teaspoons soft margarine
1 teaspoon flour	3 teaspoons flour
1 teaspoon lemon juice	1 tablespoon lemon juice

Cooking time: 20 minutes

Wash fish, cook in milk for 5 minutes until barely cooked. Lift out to skin, flake and check carefully for bones. Add beans to pan, cook until tender. Mash margarine and flour to a paste, stir briskly into pan to thicken sauce, then add fish and lemon juice.

CAULIFLOWER CHEESE

1 portion	*For freezing*
1–2 pieces cauliflower	4–6 pieces cauliflower
⅛–¼ pint (75–150 ml) milk	½ pint (300 ml) milk
1 teaspoon soft margarine	1 tablespoon soft margarine
1 teaspoon wholemeal flour	1 tablespoon wholemeal flour
2 tablespoons grated cheese	8 tablespoons grated cheese

Cooking time: 15 minutes

Cook cauliflower in milk until tender. Mash margarine and flour to paste, stir in briskly to thicken sauce, then bring to boil, and stir in cheese.

MINCED BEEF WITH SWEDE AND CARROT

1 portion	*For freezing*
2 oz (60 g) lean minced beef	½ lb (225 g) lean minced beef
1 teaspoon wholemeal flour	1 tablespoon wholemeal flour
Few slices carrot	Few slices carrot
Small piece swede	¼ lb (115 g) swede
¼ pint (150 ml) water	½ pint (300 ml) water

Cooking time: 25 minutes

Fry lean mince slowly without added fat. Stir in flour, add chopped vegetables and water, cover, and simmer gently for 20 minutes.

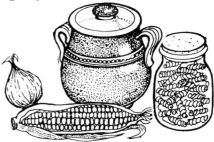

SOFT HERRING ROE WITH CABBAGE AND APPLE

1 portion	*For freezing*
1 tablespoon chopped white cabbage	4 tablespoons chopped white cabbage
1 small apple	2 medium apples
1 small soft herring roe	2–3 small soft herring roes
2–3 tablespoons water	1/4 pint (150 ml) water

Cooking time: 10–15 minutes

Place cabbage with peeled chopped apple in pan, top with washed herring roe, spoon over water. Cover and cook gently until cabbage is tender.

HAM WITH LENTILS

1 portion	*For freezing*
2 oz (60 g) lean ham or gammon	1/2 lb (225 g) lean ham or gammon
1/8–1/4 pint (75–150 ml) water	1/2 pint (300 ml) water
1 tablespoon red lentils	6 tablespoons red lentils

Cooking time: 20–30 minutes

Chop meat and cook with water and lentils in covered pan until meat is tender and lentils soft.

EGG WITH SPINACH AND BREAD

1 portion	*For freezing*
Few leaves spinach	Very good handful spinach
1–2 tablespoons milk	1/4 pint (150 ml) milk
1 tablespoon wholemeal breadcrumbs	6 tablespoons wholemeal breadcrumbs
1 egg	4 eggs

Cooking time: 10 minutes

Wash spinach well and roughly chop. Place while still wet in pan, cover, and cook gently until tender. Add milk, breadcrumbs and beaten egg, and stir gently to a scrambled texture.

One-pot two-course 'steamed' meals

A special steamer is not needed. A small cup covered with foil or boil-in-the-bag can be set in the pan alongside other food. Foods should be mashed or puréed after cooking, according to age, with extra boiled water added to achieve required consistency.

CHICKEN WITH PARSNIP AND RICE	APRICOT PURÉE
1 small joint chicken	3–4 fresh apricots
1/2 pint (300 ml) water	
1 tablespoon brown rice	
1/2 small parsnip	

Cooking time: 40 minutes

Place chicken, water and rice in pan, cover and cook for 20 minutes. Add peeled chopped parsnip, and the apricots in a well covered cup or boil-in-the-bag. Continue to cook a further 20 minutes or until all is tender. Dice and bone chicken, boil contents of pan fast to reduce cooking liquid if too wet.

FISH, POTATO AND PEAS	EGG CUSTARD
1 small potato	1/4 pint (150 ml) milk
1 small piece white fish	1 egg
1 tablespoon peas	
1 teaspoon chopped parsley	

Cooking time: 12–15 minutes

Scrub and dice potato. Bring custard milk to boil in a pan and pour half onto beaten egg in a cup. Add potato to remainder of milk and simmer 4–5 minutes. Cover cup of custard with foil, and set in pan with potato, white fish and peas alongside. Tightly cover pan and simmer gently for 7 minutes or until custard is just set. Lift out. Remove skin and bones of fish, check potato is cooked, combine vegetables with fish and parsley, adding more milk or water if liquid in pan is too reduced.

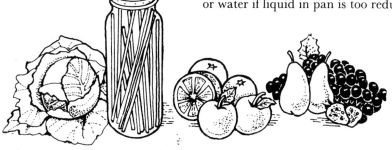

KIDNEY, CARROT AND PASTA

1 lamb's kidney
1 carrot
½–1 tablespoon wholemeal pasta
¼ pint (150 ml) water

Cooking time: 15 minutes

Halve and snip core out of kidney, remove skin. Peel and slice carrot, and put both in pan with pasta and water. Place peeled sliced apple, honey and lemon juice in covered cup or boil-in-the-bag. Put in pan, cover all and simmer gently until pasta is cooked and carrot tender.

APPLE PURÉE

1 cooking apple
1 teaspoon honey
1 teaspoon lemon juice

CAULIFLOWER DHAL

¼–⅓ pint (150–200 ml) water
2 tablespoons red lentils
1–2 sprigs cauliflower
1 tablespoon chopped watercress

Cooking time: 20–30 minutes

Grate rind and squeeze juice of orange. Separate yolk and white of egg. Whisk white to a snow, whisk in sugar until stiff. Use same whisk to whisk orange juice, yolk, margarine, flour and milk to a smooth paste. Fold two mixtures together and cover with foil in two small pots or cups (large baby food jars are ideal). Set in pan with water, lentils and sprigs of cauliflower, cover and cook for 20–30 minutes until pudding is spongy and set and lentils are soft. Add finely chopped watercress to the cauliflower dhal. There will be enough for two puddings for most babies; leave one to cool still covered and store in refrigerator until next day or freeze for later.

ORANGE PUDDING

1 small orange
1 egg
1 teaspoon brown sugar
1 teaspoon soft margarine
1 teaspoon brown flour
2 tablespoons milk

Leftover Fruit Purées

Making tiny quantities is often impractical. Make larger quantities which will purée more easily in machine.

- Freeze remainder in ice cubes.
- Add to family desserts – yogurt, custard, cream, evaporated milk or milk shake.
- Turn into jelly – ¾ pint (450 ml) liquid to 1 sachet gelatine or add to packet jelly.
- Use for fillings for flans, pies, tarts, turnovers.
- Put on a topping of crumble or sponge for family dessert.
- Use as a sauce for meat or fish – apple, apricot, gooseberry, plum, peach, pineapple for pork, gammon, sausages, herrings in oatmeal, hot or cold smoked mackerel.
- Stir into meat stews, casseroles and curries.

Leftover Vegetable Purées

- Can be frozen for later use.
- Stir in stock, water or milk to make a soup for mother's lunch.
- Stir into stews and casseroles to thicken sauces.
- Beat in egg yolk and fold in beaten egg white, bake for a quick soufflé for toddler's tea or mother's lunch.
- Add to yogurt for a salad dressing or to white sauces for more interesting topping for other vegetables to serve with a meal.
- Purées of leek, onion, cauliflower, parsnip, courgette are excellent served with lamb and pork.
- A good pancake filling for a supper dish.

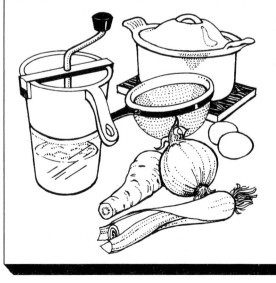

Lunch-time recipes for mother and baby

Turn baby's purée into an appetising lunch for yourself – kill two birds with one stone!

FISH CHOWDER (Purée/Soup)

1 fillet of plaice
1 small onion
1 teaspoon butter or soft margarine
1 potato, diced
3–4 tablespoons sweetcorn
Bay leaf
1 cup milk
1 teaspoon cornflour
1–1½ cups water

Cooking time: 20 minutes

Wash fish. Chop onion and fry in fat until golden. Add potato, sweetcorn, bay leaf, milk, and set fish on top. Cover and simmer 10 minutes. Lift out fish and bay leaf, discard bay leaf, fish skin and bones. Meanwhile leave chowder to cook a few more minutes. Return flaked fish to pan. ***Set aside portion for baby.*** Mix cornflour with water and thicken remainder for soup, seasoning to taste for your own lunch. Serve with sliced wholemeal bread.

CHICKEN LIVER AND TOMATO (Purée/Toast-Topper)

1 rasher lean bacon
3–4 tomatoes
2–3 chicken livers
½ teaspoon dried oregano, marjoram or basil
3–4 tablespoons water
Wholemeal bread

Chop bacon in large pieces, and fry without fat until crisp and golden. Meanwhile scald tomatoes, peel and thickly slice. Lift out bacon and keep hot. Fry chicken livers briskly on each side to colour lightly. Add tomatoes and herbs. Simmer 1–2 minutes. Pour little boiling water on small piece (¼–½ slice) of bread. ***Set aside portion for baby***, adding to it the soaked crumbled bread. Add bacon and seasoning for your own toast-topper.

BACON AND LENTIL (Purée/Soup)

2–3 rashers lean bacon
1 apple
1 small onion (optional)
4 tablespoons red lentils
2 cups water
2–3 tomatoes

Cooking time: 20–30 minutes

Dice bacon and cook gently in pan until fat runs. Peel and dice apple and onion (if used). Add to pan and fry until bacon, onion and apples are golden. Add lentils, 1 cup of water and halved tomatoes. Cover and cook gently for 20–30 minutes, lift out tomato skins, then purée. ***Set aside portion for baby.*** Add remaining water to purée and season to taste for your own lunch.

CHICKEN, CARROT AND PEAS (Purée/Toast-Topper)

1 chicken joint
1 cup water
½ teaspoon dried thyme or rosemary
1 large carrot
2–3 tablespoons frozen peas
3–5 tablespoons top of the milk
1 teaspoon cornflour

Cooking time: 40 minutes

Place chicken in pan with water and herbs, cover and simmer gently for 20–25 minutes. Meanwhile peel and dice carrot, add to pan and after 10–15 minutes' cooking, add peas. Simmer further 5–10 minutes until chicken is well cooked. Take up chicken and cut off bone into dice. Return to pan. Combine milk and cornflour. ***Set aside portion for baby*** before or after thickening cooking liquid with milk and cornflour. Season for your own toast-topper lunch.

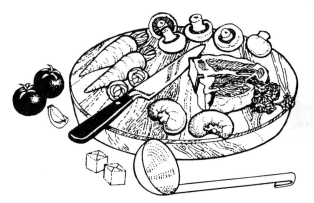

Salads for baby and family

To find salads for baby's meal that are easy to eat and digest needs a little imagination. Using some cooked vegetables in salad and moistening with yogurt when necessary will help you serve foods interesting to adults and adaptable for a baby. Give food cold, unless firmly rejected. The sooner your baby is used to foods arriving at varied temperatures the better; if you always give food warm he will be very set in his ways by twelve months, and then it could take you many *years* to persuade him to be more adventurous. The following salads should serve two parents and one to two infants.

ORANGE, CHICORY AND COTTAGE CHEESE SALAD

1 head chicory
2 carrots
2 oranges
½ lb (225 g) carton cottage cheese
3 tablespoons French dressing

Wash chicory and separate leaves. Cut carrots into big matchsticks and lightly cook in very little water until tender and water has evaporated. Coarsely grate a little orange rind. Then peel and cut orange into segments. Arrange chicory round dish then set cheese in centre, toss orange rind and flesh with carrot in French dressing and pile in centre of dish.
Baby note: Purée finely chopped chicory, combine all remaining items without dressing until ten months, then dressing optional.

EGGS HONGROISE

½ lb (225 g) frozen sweetcorn
¼ lb (115 g) frozen peas
6 hard-boiled eggs, sliced
1 onion
4 tablespoons sunflower or corn oil
1–2 teaspoons mild paprika
1–2 tablespoons vinegar
1 red pepper, or small tin pimento

Cook corn and peas together. Place at bottom of dish, cover with hard-boiled eggs. Chop onion and fry gently in oil with paprika (do not allow to brown). Add vinegar, spoon over egg dish and top with sliced cooked red pepper or tinned pimento.
Baby note: Serve to baby before adding dressing.

CHICKEN SALAD NIÇOISE

½ cooked cold chicken
3 tablespoons yogurt
1 tablespoon tomato purée
1 teaspoon marjoram or basil
½ lb (225 g) cooked green beans or peas
¼ cucumber
Few anchovies and black olives (optional)
3 large tomatoes

Dice chicken, toss in yogurt, tomato purée, herbs and seasoning. Place in bottom of dish. Top with cooked beans or peas. Cover with sliced cucumber. Decorate with anchovies and olives. Surround dish with skinned tomatoes (plunge into water when cooking beans or peas for 8 seconds).
Baby note: Reserve baby's chicken in yogurt before adding salt or pepper. Combine with beans and mashed tomato. Give cucumber after eight to twelve months.

BEEF ITALIEN

1 aubergine
1–2 tablespoons sunflower or corn oil
1 tablespoon chopped fresh parsley (or marjoram)
1 onion, chopped
1 green pepper, sliced
Home-cooked cold beef
1 small carton soured cream

Slice but do not peel aubergine, sprinkle with salt and leave to drain out indigestible juices for 30 minutes. Rinse off salt, and pat dry. Fry aubergine in oil until brown on one side, cover pan and cook gently until soft. Add herbs, season with salt and pepper. Cook onion and pepper in pan of fast boiling water until tender, but not mushy. Drain and cool. Cut meat in fingers. Toss all together and dot with soured cream.
Baby note: For over eight months, mince or dice meat and combine with vegetables. Use only a little soured cream.

Adapting family meals for baby

Many traditional favourite meals can be adapted so that some of the food may be given to your baby. Feed baby before or during the family meal. If he has his meal after yours, set his portion on one side at lunch, cover, but do not keep hot. No need to boil food before serving just one or two hours after a family meal. Re-heat quickly if preferred warm in a small plate over a pan of boiling water, or in a microwave oven, whichever is convenient. Food will lose Vitamin C if kept hot.

Where possible avoid adding salt to foods until baby's portion has been set on one side. This is important for under eight months.

Cottage Pie, Carrots
Sponge Pudding, Custard

Baby: Cottage pie, carrots puréed or mashed. Custard with mashed banana.

Spaghetti Bolognese
Green Salad
Blackberry and Apple Crumble

Baby: Spaghetti, bolognese sauce and a little salad puréed with or without dressing. Apple (omit blackberries) and crumble topping.

Roast Pork, Apple Sauce
Sage and Onion Stuffing
Parsnips, Sprouts, Roast Potatoes
Lemon Meringue Pie

Baby: Stuffing, parsnip, sprouts, inside of roast potatoes and Cheddar or cottage cheese puréed together. Serve apple sauce for pudding.

Stew, Jacket Potatoes, Peas
Rice Pudding

Baby: Give stew, inside of potatoes and peas, puréed. Give rice pudding.

Steak and Kidney Pie
Mashed Potatoes, Cabbage
Fruit Salad and Ice Cream

Baby: Steak, kidney and gravy, no pastry – plus potato and cabbage, puréed. Fruit salad – avoid sweet syrup – with little or no ice cream.

Fish and Chips
Mushy Peas
Fruit Yogurt

Baby: Mushy peas and steamed or poached fish/scrambled egg/cottage or Cheddar cheese. No chips or fish in batter. Plain yogurt with finely grated apple, pear or mashed banana.

Lasagne, Salad
Ice Cream

Baby: Lasagne (if not too oily) puréed with salad or mashed with *very* finely chopped salad items. Ice cream only if home-made from fruit purée, eggs and evaporated milk; if cream is used give only small portion.

Beef Curry
Dhal (Lentil Purée)
Brown Rice, Tomato
Banana Raita
(Sliced Bananas in Plain Yogurt)
Stewed or Fresh Fruit

Baby: Lentil purée, brown rice, tomato and banana raita. Give stewed or fresh fruit.

Mixed Grill
Chips, Salad
Apple Pie, Custard

Baby: Include liver or kidney in grill, plus tomatoes for easy purée, adding a little instant cereal and boiled water. No chips. Give apple and custard without pastry topping.

Roast Chicken
Cauliflower in White Sauce
Roast Potatoes, Stuffing, Gravy
Mousse

Baby: Chicken without skin, cauliflower and sauce, centre of potato or stuffing, purée with gravy. Only give home-made mousses made with eggs, evaporated milk and fruit purée. Omit dessert entirely if not suitable and give larger portion of main course or fresh fruit.

Improve your favourite recipes

The recipes in this section are basically familiar favourites popular with young children. All have been very specially designed to ensure that they have maximum nutritional value, as so many nutrients are lost by other methods of cookery. With these as a guide you can adapt your own favourite family recipes and ensure they too provide the best for your children, keeping sugar and fat to a minimum, vitamins, minerals and fibre high.

The soup and casserole recipes may be made early in the day to re-heat separately for childrens' tea and adults' evening meal. Similarly, the supper pies, cheap and convenient, can be prepared for tea, with adult portions left ready for later. Serve the pies with freshly cooked green vegetables or salad.

The recipes will serve two adults and two small children.

FARMHOUSE VEGETABLE SOUP

1 tablespoon oil
1 onion, chopped
1 large carrot, chopped
2 sticks celery, chopped
1 potato
1¼ pints (750 ml) chicken stock
1 bay leaf
1 teaspoon mixed herbs
3 sprouts or two outer cabbage leaves, finely shredded
2 tomatoes
Grated cheese

Heat oil in large pan and add onion, carrot and celery. Cook until golden. Add diced scrubbed (*not* peeled) potato, stock, bay leaf and herbs. Cover and simmer for 10 minutes. Add greens and simmer a further 10 minutes. Season to taste adding chopped tomato. Serve well sprinkled with cheese, with a slice of bread.

CARROT AND ORANGE SOUP

1 lb (450 g) carrots
1 onion
1¼ pints (750 ml) chicken stock
1 cup orange juice

Slice carrot and onion, and simmer in chicken stock until very tender. Purée to a fine velvety texture. Stir in orange juice when reheating just before serving.

FISH AND WATERCRESS SOUP

1 large whiting, filleted (but keep bone)
1¾ pints (1 litre) water
1 bay leaf
1 tablespoon oil
1 onion, sliced
1 medium potato, sliced
1 bunch watercress, chopped
6 tablespoons dried milk powder
1–2 tablespoons mayonnaise (optional)

Wash fish and fish bone, and place in pan with water and bay leaf. Simmer 10 minutes then turn all into bowl. Heat oil and fry slices of onion and potato, covered, slowly without browning. Pour on fish stock and simmer for 7–10 minutes or until potato is cooked. Add watercress, simmer for 2–3 minutes, then add flaked, boned fish. Purée soup with milk powder, or it may be left rough if preferred. Add mayonnaise to soup bowls. Extra dried milk may be added for children.

FISH PIE

1 lb (450 g) potatoes
1 lb (450 g) coley or other white fish
½ lb (225 g) frozen peas
½ pint (300 ml) milk
1½ oz (45 g) soft margarine
1 rounded tablespoon flour
2 tablespoons chopped parsley
1 hard-boiled egg, chopped
3 tablespoons dried milk powder

Peel and boil potatoes. Meanwhile, wash fish and place in separate pan with peas and milk. Bring to boil and simmer 5 minutes. Tip all into pie dish. Melt margarine in used pan, add flour, stir to blend then remove from heat. Blend in the milk from the fish and peas. Beat until smooth, then bring to the boil. Remove from heat and add parsley, seasoning and hard-boiled egg. Remove skin and bone from fish. Pour sauce over fish and peas and fold together. Drain the cooked potatoes, reserving water. Mash, adding powdered milk and sufficient potato water for a soft, creamy texture. Top pies with potato, making a separate fish pie (or pies) for childrens' tea if they eat earlier than adults, and reheat in oven to serve.

COWBOY PIE WITH CORN

½ lb (225 g) lean minced beef
1 rounded tablespoon oatmeal
¼ pint (150 ml) water
1 lb (450 g) potatoes
1 medium can baked beans
4 oz (115 g) sweetcorn

Fry mince slowly without adding fat. Stir well until meat becomes crumbly and the fat runs. Add oatmeal and water. Cover and cook very gently for 15–20 minutes. Meanwhile peel and boil potatoes in a little water. Stir beans and corn into mince. Simmer 3–4 minutes. Turn into pie dish and top with potatoes well mashed with dried milk and some of their cooking water. Brown under grill if wished.

SHEPHERDS CARROT CRUMBLE

¾ lb (350 g) cold roast lamb or beef
1 onion, sliced
2 tablespoons oil
2 tablespoons flour
½ pint (300 ml) stock
1 tablespoon tomato purée
1 lb (450 g) carrots, sliced
2 oz (60 g) soft margarine
1 teaspoon dried rosemary or thyme
4 oz (115 g) wholemeal flour
1 teacup fresh breadcrumbs

Oven temperature: 190°C/375°F/Gas 5
Mince or finely chop meat, discarding fat. Cook onion in oil until golden, then stir in flour. Cook a further 1–2 minutes to colour lightly, then add stock, purée and carrots. Bring to boil then cover and cook slowly for 10 minutes. Remove from heat and add meat, season and turn into serving dishes. Rub fat into herbs, wholemeal flour and breadcrumbs and scatter over meat. Bake 30 minutes.

DEVONSHIRE BEEF AND POTATO PIE

1 lb (450 g) potatoes
½ lb (225 g) swede
1 onion
¾ lb (350 g) braising steak
¾ pint (425 ml) stock (approx.)

Oven temperature: 180°C/350°F/Gas 4
Thinly slice potato, swede, onion and meat. Arrange in layers in ovenproof dish, finishing with potato. Pour over enough boiling stock to almost reach top of potatoes. Cover with lid or oiled foil. Bake 1½ hours. Remove lid and brown for further half hour.

SAUSAGE AND GREEN BEAN PIE

1 lb (450 g) sausagemeat
1 lb (450 g) sliced green beans
1 lb (450 g) potatoes
1 tablespoon soft margarine
1 tablespoon flour
⅓ pint (200 ml) milk
Nutmeg
3 tablespoons dried milk
2 tablespoons grated cheese

Oven temperature: 190°C/375°F/Gas 5
Pat out sausagemeat in 1 or 2 small, well-floured pie dishes with floured or wet fingers to cover base. Bake for 30 minutes and drain off any fat (do not worry if meat has shrunk or looks misshapen). Cook beans and potatoes separately. Melt margarine in saucepan, then stir in flour and milk. Season with salt, pepper and nutmeg, and fold in drained green beans. Put onto sausagemeat, and top with potatoes, well mashed with dried milk and a little of their cooking liquid. Sprinkle with cheese, grill and serve, or reheat by baking for half an hour.

CHICKEN LOUISE

3 chicken joints
¾ pint (425 ml) water
1 teaspoon dried rosemary
3 large carrots, sliced
3½ oz (100 g) pasta shells or shapes
7 oz (200 g) broad beans
3 tablespoons dried milk
1 rounded tablespoon soft margarine
1 rounded tablespoon flour
1 tablespoon chopped parsley
2 tablespoons lemon juice

Put chicken in pan with water and rosemary, and simmer for 35 minutes. Add carrots, pasta shells and broad beans. Simmer for a further 12 minutes or until everything is cooked. Stir in milk powder. Blend margarine and flour to a smooth paste and stir into casserole to thicken juices. Add parsley and lemon juice, and season to taste.

CHICKEN AND LEEK PILAFF

3 chicken joints
3 medium leeks
1 tablespoon oil
1 cup brown rice
1½ cups chicken stock
1 bay leaf
1 teaspoon oregano
3½ oz (100 g) raisins

Cut meat from chicken bones, and use the bones and skin to make stock. Cut leeks in 2 inch (5 cm) lengths. Fry chicken in hot oil, then add rice and leeks. Pour on stock and herbs and season. Cover well and simmer for 30 minutes. Add raisins and a little water if stock is already absorbed. Cook for a further 10–15 minutes until rice is tender.

SAUSAGE AND KIDNEY CASSEROLE

6 lamb's kidneys
6–8 chipolata sausages
1 onion
1 tablespoon oil (optional)
1 tablespoon flour
1 medium tin tomatoes

Halve, skin and core kidneys. Fry sausages gently until fat runs, then lift out of pan. Fry kidney cut side up quickly, and turn once. Add oil if needed, then stir in first flour, then tomatoes. Halve sausages and return to pan. Cover all and simmer on top of cooker or in oven for 10–15 minutes.

RABBIT AND BACON CASSEROLE

3 rashers streaky bacon
3–4 joints rabbit
1–2 onions
1 tablespoon flour
1/2 pint (300 ml) stock
2 teaspoons tomato purée
1 bay leaf
1/2 lb (225 g) new or small potatoes

Oven temperature, if used: 180°C/350°F/Gas 4
Halve and fry rashers of bacon. Cook until brown, lift out and set to one side. Add rabbit and quartered onions. Fry until brown then stir in flour, stock, tomato purée and bay leaf. Add potatoes then cover and simmer for 50–60 minutes.

PORK AND BEAN CASSEROLE

1/4 lb (115 g) red kidney beans
1 lb (450 g) lean belly pork
1 tablespoon flour
1/2 tablespoon mild paprika
1/2 pint (300 ml) liquid from soaking beans
3 tablespoons tomato purée

Soak beans by pouring on boiling water, and leave overnight. Trim skin off pork and fry until golden in its own fat. Stir in flour and paprika, and cook for 1–2 minutes without browning. Add measured liquid from beans, as well as beans and tomato purée. Cook for 1–1 1/4 hours.

LANCASHIRE HOT POT

1 1/2 lb (700 g) pieces of lean middle neck lamb
1 onion, sliced
1 tablespoon flour
1/2 pint (300 ml) water or stock
2 lamb's kidneys
1/4 lb (115 g) mushrooms
1 lb (450 g) potatoes

Oven temperature: 180°C/350°F/Gas 4
Brown meat in own fat until golden. Add onion to pan and cook until golden. Place both in ovenproof casserole. Stir flour and liquid together, then pour over meat. Add cleaned, sliced kidney and mushrooms, and season with salt and pepper. Cover with scrubbed, thinly sliced potatoes. Cover and bake 1 hour then uncover and cook for a further 20 minutes to brown the top.

HAM WITH BROAD BEANS AND PASTA SHELLS

6–8 oz (175–225 g) thick sliced ham
1/2 lb (225 g) broad beans
1/4 lb (115 g) pasta shells
1 tablespoon parsley
3 tablespoons French dressing
2 tablespoons cream or yogurt

Cut ham into fingers. Cook beans and pasta separately until tender. Drain both and rinse briefly under cold water to prevent pasta sticking together. Toss both together in parsley, dressing and cream or yogurt. Leave to cool, season before adding ham.

This makes a light lunch or a tasty cold starter.

STUFFED EGG MAYONNAISE

1/2 cauliflower
1 bunch watercress
4 hard-boiled eggs
1/4 lb (115 g) low-fat curd cheese
6 tablespoons mayonnaise (good bought or home-made)

Cook cauliflower sprigs until tender, and drain. Chop *stalks* of washed watercress, and toss with cauliflower and arrange in bottom of dish. Halve eggs. Press three-quarters of yolks through a sieve, and bind with curd cheese and a little mayonnaise to soften. Season to taste. Sandwich egg whites with this filling, set on vegetables. Spoon mayonnaise over and sprinkle on remaining sieved yolk. Garnish with the watercress leaves.

Serve as a starter, or to accompany another salad meal.

Puddings

Most of us have grown up with the idea that puddings are part of every main meal, but nutritionally many of them are very poor, being high in fat, sugar and refined starches. Usually they are eaten by small children at the expense of the protein and vegetable course eaten before. Once infants accept that every first course is always followed by a pudding, many will readily forego the main dish, knowing they are not really hungry enough for both, and they may even get second helpings of pudding after only toying with the main dish.

For children under seven and most adults the calorie requirements are small and are often exceeded, causing overweight. During the period when young children are growing up, the family pudding course – if it is served – should aim at providing fruit foremost, or milk and eggs. Dishes that contribute little – treacle tart, jam roly poly, chocolate sponge, meringues with cream, lemon meringue pie – should be avoided. Few but manual workers and teenagers can eat these plus all the nutrients they require without being overweight. Children under three years are undergoing the very important period of brain growth. Many are notoriously difficult to feed because their calorie requirements are low, thus they are very easily satisfied by foods high in calories. If the foods given are low in their nutritional requirements their health and intellect could suffer. Ensure any puddings given do provide useful nutrients.

Two-course meals are undoubtedly more interesting and enjoyable, but the course other than the main one of meat and vegetables need *not* be a pudding. Many vegetables that are unpopular served as vegetables can be very popular as soups with the texture considerably changed or combined with other vegetables to mask their flavour. Try leek and potato, parsnip, carrot and orange, tomato and lentil, creamed apple and spinach. These make an excellent first course and can be used for baby, packed meals, or mother's lunch too.

Alternative first courses can be based on salads and fruits. Avocado with grapes, celery with apple and raisins, melon with cucumber and tomato. Diced items can be tossed together or set in piles on a toddler's plate with a French, yogurt or cream cheese dressing handed round for those who want it.

Where a low protein main dish is served – cauliflower or macaroni cheese, for instance – a useful starter would be hot wholemeal bread with a pâté or spread of liver, sardine or other fish, or nuts. It is a French custom to serve a vegetable dish separately from the meat course and some hot vegetable dishes lend themselves well to being used to start a meal. Broad beans and carrots in parsley sauce; courgettes and onions in tomato sauce; onion and Jerusalem artichokes and potatoes in a mushroom sauce, cooked asparagus or globe artichokes – may all be served before the main dish, and thus the pudding can be omitted.

Nutritious puddings

Choose those based on fruit and milk, keep sugar to a minimum, and where favourite recipes call for flour, use wholemeal or a brown flour or a combination of brown and white in the recipe.

Fruit crumble: Have plenty of fruit at the bottom without sugar if possible. One part soft margarine, one or two parts brown sugar, three parts flour and three parts wholemeal breadcrumbs for topping; with cup as measure, you will have plenty to freeze for later. With tablespoon as measure, enough for one dessert.

Fruit salads: Combine two to four fruits using fresh, frozen, dried or canned fruits (preferably in fruit juice, not syrup). Good combinations are:
Cooked rhubarb and raspberries
Mandarins and banana
Pears and black grapes
Stewed apples and raisins
Pineapple, orange and banana

Fruit pies: Keep pastry to a minimum, roll very thin and have plenty of fruit filling. *Avoid* packet or tinned pie fillings – they have much less food value than home-made fillings which are free of modified starch filler, artificial colour and flavour.

Baked fruit: Apples stuffed with dates and honey
Apple stuffed with raisins and orange rind
Bananas with orange juice
Rhubarb with redcurrant jelly
Apricots stoned and stuffed with almond paste
Peaches with orange juice
Pears with cinnamon and red wine, cider, Ribena or apple juice
Apples in pure apple juice

Fruit jellies: Any thin purées of fruit and fruit juice (tinned, jars or cartons) can be turned into a jelly. These are much more nutritious than commercial jellies. Place 4 tablespoons cold water in a small pan, sprinkle on a sachet gelatine, and leave to soak 1 minute. Heat very gently to melt crystals without boiling, and when dissolved add cold (but not chilled) ¾ pint (425 ml) juice or purée. Pour into container to set. (Pineapple juices are sometimes temperamental with gelatine. Boil juice to kill enzymes if jelly does not set, and add a further sachet of gelatine.)

Fruit with yogurt: Use plain yogurt with fruit, or use fruit or nut yogurts as a dressing on fresh, frozen or tinned fruits for a fruitier dessert. Commercial fruit yogurts are very sweet and have strong artificial flavours which tend to spoil a child's palate for real foods so, if used, they should be combined with fresh, frozen or unsweetened tinned fruits to redress the balance. (It is always easy, though, to make your *own* fruit yogurts.)
Good combinations are:
Grapes and pear with plain yogurt
 – grilled sugar topping
Banana with orange yogurt
Pears with blackcurrant yogurt
Peaches with Melba or raspberry
 yogurt
Apples with lemon yogurt
Apples and raisins with muesli
 yogurt
Apricots and pears with hazelnut
 yogurt.

Accompaniments for fruit desserts: Cream is high in animal fat, and synthetic alternatives are possibly no healthier. Good toppings are evaporated milk or plain yogurt. Combine the two if you wish and also try Cremet (equal quantities of yogurt and cold custard with or without whipped cream or evaporated milk).

Milk puddings: Custard and rice puddings are popular with many children and provide useful extra milk in the diet. Custard can be home-made from egg, flour and vanilla essence for those who need an additive-free diet; add only as much sugar as you wish. Tinned rice puddings are not very heavily sweetened; the main food value is the milk content, as the polished rice provides little value. No artificial flavour or colour usually added, so this may be a useful dessert. Most instant desserts where you just add milk are sickeningly sweet and highly artificially flavoured; they spoil your child's palate for real foods and are best used only if there is really no other way your child can be persuaded to take milk.

Chapter Five
Troublesome toddlers

The appetite and calorie requirements quite often drop at some stage in a child's second year. Children grow at their slowest rate between fifteen months and four years, so it is not surprising that the demand for food becomes less urgent. By one year many toddlers are being moved to an adult diet which is quite high in disguised fat, sugar and starches and adds many more calories to food than the more carefully chosen fruit and vegetable purées and other foods of the first year.

What Causes the Troubles
(calories per 1 oz or 27 g)

Appetite Killers	Calories
Butter and other fats	200–250
Chocolate and crisps	165
Can of Coke or pop	150
Sweet and chocolate biscuits	140
Cake	120–140
Sweets	110+
Instant dessert powder	105
Sausages (pork)	100
Chips	70

Nutritious Food and Snacks	Calories
Fish finger, liver	50
8 fl. oz (225 ml) drink, ½ orange juice, ½ water	50
Egg	42
Jacket potato, kidney	25
Banana	22
Milk	19
Baked beans	17
Apple	13
Carrot	6

In order to maintain a healthy diet for this age group, who still have high nutritional requirements, it is important to largely or completely omit foods which contain a high proportion of fat, sugar or refined starches. Sweets, chocolate, pop, crisps, iced cakes and biscuits in particular should be *very* limited; also instant puddings, pastries and chips. Once all these foods are introduced into the diet of a one- to two-year-old they can very quickly become the major part of his intake with foods of real value largely squeezed out.

The junk food syndrome

After carefully chosen baby foods, toddlers can very quickly slip into a diet of manufactured foods. The colours, textures and flavours have been designed to beguile; and the content of chemical additives, colour, flavourings, anti-oxidants, stabilisers, preservatives etc. is extraordinarily high in relation to the content of 'real food'. Some foods lose many nutrients in the processing and gain many chemicals; a diet of these products will lead to vitamin, mineral and sometimes protein deficiencies, and the chemicals may also cause emotional disorders similar to hyperactivity. Some chemicals considered 'safe' in one country are banned in another, and it is, anyway, unlikely that they have been sufficiently tested in the combinations as well as quantities of a toddler's diet. Some can damage the nutritional value of foods, putting toddlers at greater risk of nutritional deficiencies.

Sadly, about 5 oz (130 g) sugar is now the average daily consumption of many young children. This provides one-half to one-third of the calories a child under seven requires. As a result most children consume far less than they need in protein, vitamins and minerals or, conversely, in order to consume enough of these, take too many calories and risk overweight. Children whose diet is deficient in protein, more especially vitamins and minerals, will show a variety of ailments. If the B vitamins are limited in the diet, the child's personality will be affected, causing irritability, depression, aggression, sleeplessness and poor appetite. This combined with a high intake of sodium (salt in crisps and on other foods) and a low intake of potassium (fruit and vegetables) also causes lethargy and fatigue. The high consumption of refined starch, sugar and salt puts a great strain on the production of insulin from the pancreas and hormones from the adrenal glands which may cause long-term damage to the health.

Highly sweetened foods are quickly converted into sugar in the blood and so give a short burst of energy. This will be quickly used and then fatigue will follow as the blood sugar level drops. Topping up with sweet food every hour quickly becomes a habit to keep them going and prevent the tiredness and bad temper that results from the drop in blood sugar level. Some foods are digested much more slowly and a steady supply is therefore converted for energy. Fat, protein and carbohydrates from grains and root vegetables (bread, flour, breakfast cereal, rice, pasta, potato, carrots etc.) are slowly converted so that a gap of three to five hours can be allowed where these foods are eaten. Fibre in the diet further slows the conversion process so is also very useful. Where only a small quantity of sugar is consumed at meals, and meals carefully chosen, the temperament of a toddler will be much more even; he is likely to be more equable, cooperative and easier to manage.

Faddy toddlers

Between eighteen months and two years infants become much more acutely aware of the tastes and textures of their food. In some families there is normally a much greater awareness or consciousness of what they eat, while in other families there is less concern with varied tastes and textures; food is gobbled down cheerfully by all. Patience is needed to gently accustom your child to the varied tastes and textures. If a good variety of foods were given in the early, less conservative days it is usually easier to cope with toddlers later.

Disguising tastes and textures is a good plan to make a wider range of foods more acceptable. Use mixer, blender or mashers and combine foods to alter flavours. Leek and tomato soup puréed should be called 'tomato soup' if leeks are not popular.

Parsnips, swede and turnip can be mashed and well masked by potato purée. Bolognese sauce with celery, onion, liver, mince and tomatoes can be puréed to prevent picky children fussing about contents.

The toddler stage is also one in which they develop an awareness of relationships. Babies usually want only to please a parent while many a little bit older have developed quite a will of their own and realise they can either please themselves or please a parent. Meal- and bed-times are occasions when they can be particularly difficult to manage as they learn how their own behaviour can affect yours. Try to avoid head-on battles wherever possible but do not allow your toddler to lead you a song and dance. Get on with some other job if he is unwilling to cooperate at meal times; you will then not feel frustrated yourself and that you are wasting your time. It will also be easier for you to be patient and cheerful. You may not be able to control your child's temperament and whims but at least the control of your own is in your hands and that is half the battle; when *his* extreme behaviour does not gain much response from you, he is unlikely to try it for long.

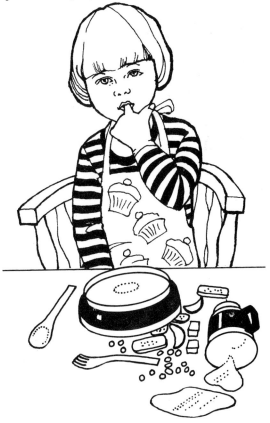

Daily nutritional requirements for 1 ½–4 year old

Calcium
Daily Requirement
500 mg

Iron
Daily Requirement
7–8 mg

Vitamin A
Daily Requirement
300 mcg

Thiamin
Daily Requirement
0.6 mg

TOTAL DAILY INTAKE PROVIDED BY ANY OF THE FOLLOWING

Calcium	Iron	Vitamin A	Thiamin
425 ml (¾ pint) milk	75 g (2½ oz) liver	7 g (¼ oz) liver	90 g (3 oz) pork
70 g (2¼ oz) Cheddar cheese	35 g (1¼ oz) black pudding	15 g (½ oz) old carrots	70 g (2¼ oz) peanuts
60 g (2 oz) sesame seed	45 g (1½ oz) Readybrek	60 g (2 oz) new carrots	30 g (1 oz) wheatgerm
		60 g (2 oz) spinach	90 g (3 oz) luncheon meat
		30 g (1 oz) Readybrek	35 g (1¼ oz) Readybrek
		30 g (1 oz) butter	15 g (½ oz) oat germ or bran
		35 g (1¼ oz) margarine	

QUARTER DAILY INTAKE PROVIDED BY ANY OF THE FOLLOWING

Calcium	Iron	Vitamin A	Thiamin
35 g (1¼ oz) sardines	60 g (2 oz) corned beef	1 egg	425 ml (¾ pint) milk
½ small carton yogurt	60 g (2 oz) kidney	300 ml (½ pint) milk	50 g (1¾ oz) chicken
55 g (1¾ oz) almonds	75 g (2½ oz) beef	30 g (1 oz) kidney	50 g (1¾ oz) kidney
45 g (1½ oz) figs	90 g (3 oz) lamb	1 large peach	45 g (1½ oz) pork sausage
60 g (2 oz) watercress	1 egg	60 g (2 oz) melon	45 g (1½ oz) bacon
425 ml (¾ pint) soya milk	75 g (2½ oz) sardines	60 g (2 oz) fresh apricots	60 g (2 oz) peanuts
	30 g (1 oz) dried haricots	15 g (½ oz) dried apricots	60 g (2 oz) liver
	20 g (¾ oz) lentils	½ carton fortified plain yogurt	90 g (3 oz) bread
	60 g (2 oz) brown bread		60 g (2 oz) peas
	115 g (4 oz) white bread	90 g (3 oz) tomatoes	1 tsp Marmite
	30 g (1 oz) iron fortified cereals	115 g (4 oz) sprouts	35 g (1¼ oz) lentils
		150 g (5 oz) baked beans	15 g (½ oz) most cereals

Required for teeth and bones. Lack causes poor healing of cuts and broken bones. Vitamin D required for absorption.

Required by blood to prevent anaemia. Vitamin C required for absorption. Many children healthy on well below recommended level if Vitamin C is taken.

Required by moist surface of eyes, throat, lungs, also skin; lack increases risk of bronchitis and infections of skin, eyes and throat.

Required for good general health and appetite.

Protein Daily Requirement 25–40 g (¾–1¼ oz) Required for growth of body and brain.

make up total grams from

575 ml (1 pint) milk	**18**	60 g (2 oz) Cheddar cheese	**14**	60 g (2 oz) fish fingers	**7**	30 g (1 oz) oats or wholewheat cereal	**3**
60 g (2 oz) lean beef	**17**			60 g (2 oz) pasta (dry)	**6**		
60 g (2 oz) peanuts	**16**	60 g (2 oz) lamb or sardines	**13**	115 g (4 oz) baked beans	**6**	60 g (2 oz) tofu	**2½**
60 g (2 oz) pork	**16**					60 g (2 oz) sprouts	**2**
60 g (2 oz) corned beef	**15**	60 g (2 oz) white fish	**10**	60 g (2 oz) sausage	**5**	25 g (1 oz) cornflakes, Rice Krispies	**1½–2**
60 g (2 oz) chicken	**14**	60 g (2 oz) kidney	**10**	60 g (2 oz) bread	**5**		
60 g (2 oz) bacon or ham	**14**	1 small carton plain yogurt	**7**	60 g (2 oz) broad beans	**4**	60 g (2 oz) potato	**1¼**
60 g (2 oz) liver	**14**	1 egg	**7**	30 g (1 oz) Readybrek	**4**		
				60 g (2 oz) peas	**3**		

Riboflavin

Daily Requirement
0.7–0.8 mg

Nicotinic Acid

Daily Requirement
Niacin 8–9 mg

Vitamin C

Daily Requirement
20 mg

Vitamin D

Daily requirement
10 mcg

TOTAL DAILY INTAKE PROVIDED BY ANY OF THE FOLLOWING

Riboflavin	Nicotinic Acid	Vitamin C	Vitamin D
45 g (1½ oz) kidney	35 g (1¼ oz) liver	15 g (½ oz) blackcurrants	20 g (¾ oz) herring
20–30 g (¾–1 oz) liver	45 g (1½ oz) peanuts	60 g (2 oz) sprouts	90 g (3 oz) tinned salmon
575 ml (1 pint) milk	75 g (2½ oz) chicken	90 g (3 oz) cabbage or	60 g (2 oz) Readybrek
35 g (1¼ oz) Readybrek	75 g (2½ oz) pork	cauliflower	
45 g (1½ oz) fortified	60 g (2 oz) sardines	1 large banana	
cereals	35 g (1¼ oz) Readybrek	60 g (2 oz) citrus fruit	
30 g (1 oz) Cheddar	45 g (1½ oz) Grape Nuts	75 g (2½ oz) new potato	
cheese			

QUARTER DAILY INTAKE PROVIDED BY ANY OF THE FOLLOWING

Riboflavin	Nicotinic Acid	Vitamin C	Vitamin D
75 g (2½ oz) lamb	15 g (½ oz) most cereals	575 ml (1 pint) milk	35 g (1¼ oz) margarine
60 g (2 oz) beef	425 ml (¾ pint) milk	30 g (1 oz) peas	30 g (1 oz) liver
90 g (3 oz) bacon/pork	20 g (¾ oz) bacon	90 g (3 oz) carrots	75 g (2½ oz) Cheddar
90 g (3 oz) chicken/ham	50 g (1¾ oz) kidney	115 g (4 oz) old potatoes	cheese
1½ tbsp wheatgerm	45 g (1½ oz) beef/lamb	60 g (2 oz) kidney	30 g (1 oz) sardines
½ tsp Marmite	45 g (1½ oz) Cheddar	30 g (1 oz) liver	1 small carton fortified
½ small carton yogurt	cheese	1 medium apple	yogurt
50 g (1¾ oz) sardines	45 g (1½ oz) white fish	½ tomato	15 g (½ oz) Readybrek
90 g (3 oz) spinach	30 g (1 oz) ham/sausage	30 g (1 oz) runner beans	
1 egg	60 g (2 oz) broad beans	20 g (¾ oz) broad beans	
60 g (2 oz) sultanas	30 g (1 oz) lentils	20 g (¾ oz) gooseberries	
35 g (1¼ oz) mushrooms	1 tbsp wheatgerm	15 g (½ oz) Readybrek	
15 g (½ oz) wheatflakes	¼ tsp Marmite		
15 g (½ oz) Weetabix	¼ tsp Bovril		
	115 g (4 oz) bread		

Required for health and
growth. Lack causes poor
appetite, cracks and sores
round nose and mouth.

Required for health and
strength. Lack may cause
ulcers in mouth and poor
general health.

Required for health and
growth. Lack causes
anaemia, low resistance to
infection. Easily lost in
cooking.

Required for bones and
teeth. Some Vitamin D
manufactured in skin
exposed to sunlight.
Supplements advised but
overdose of these can
cause damage to kidneys
and brain.

Fats

15–30 g (½–1 oz)
made up of butter
or soft margarine
plus little corn or
sunflower oil
plus 575 ml (1 pint)
milk
plus 1–3 portions
meat, oily fish,

eggs, cheese or
nuts.

Some fat is essential
for absorption of
Vitamins A, D, E
and K. Diet should
be low in animal
fats which are high
in cholesterol.

Dietary fibre

1 portion wholegrain
bread or cereal
plus 1–3 portions
fruit or vegetables.

Fibre required for
proper movement
of the bowels.

Fluids

850 ml–1 litre
(1½–2 pints)
recommended
575 ml (1 pint) milk
plus 150–200 ml
(¼–⅓ pint)
diluted fruit syrup
plus 150–425 ml
(¼–¾ pint) water

Required for proper
working of kidneys,
and insufficient may
cause damage. Tea
and coffee should
not be given – they
contain strong
stimulants not
advised for young
children.

Guidelines for eating problems

DO give small portions and leave children to feed themselves; they will always ask for more if they want it. They won't behave nearly so badly if they are left to manage on their own. If they need a long time to eat a meal give it, and get on with the washing up, ironing or cleaning the cooker so that you do not lose patience.

DO make food look colourful and attractive on a plate. Serve small piles of food separately, not all mixed up, if they prefer it that way.

DO ensure children are comfortable and that the chair is the right height. Have suitable implements, and unbreakable pretty plates that they can use with ease. Do not fuss about table manners if they prefer fingers to forks when two and three years old, so long as they can manage knife, fork and spoon properly by five years when they have school lunch.

DO try to sit down as a family for most meals so that these are a pleasant social event. Choose food that will hopefully suit all, with a variety of vegetables if some are unpopular.

DO give only as many meals or snacks a day as are eaten with relish. It may be two, three or six even, but see that all are healthy and well balanced, however small.

DO give regular vitamin supplements until five or, if not eating well, seven years or more. Increase nutritional value of foods by adding extra dried milk powder to mashed potato, fruit purée, soups, drinks, custard etc. Choose breakfast cereals with high nutritional value.

DON'T force, coerce or persuade your child to eat what he is reluctant to eat or expect him to eat everything. Simply place a dish of food in front of him without comment and if he does not eat it in a reasonable amount of time take it away. Give him a small quantity of a chosen dessert; if this is not eaten make him wait until the next proper meal or snack-time. Never bribe with sweets or promises of puddings. Never make any comment on the food you give your child; that it is good for him, will make him strong, etc.

DON'T let him force, coerce or persuade you to give him food or drink you consider unsuitable. They are easily influenced by friends or TV advertising. Do not give sweets, biscuits, pop after a meal that has not been eaten; he does *not* need something to help him out until the next meal.

It is usually easier not to have in the house food you do not wish him to eat. Keep cake cut in portions in the freezer, and bring out only what *you wish* your family to eat. Just don't buy sweet biscuits, crisps and sweets, and avoid aisles in supermarkets containing forbidden foods.

DON'T give foods between meals or unplanned snack-times except in very special circumstances. If food is not eaten at meal-time make sure children learn that they will have to wait two to four hours before the next meal or planned snack, and cannot expect anything after the meal to tide them over.

DON'T give highly spiced or salted foods to children. Their sense of taste is much more sensitive than an adult's.

DON'T give more than half to one cup of liquid at meals. It will be too 'filling' for some. Give drinks between meals at snack-times largely, so quantities will not be needed at main meal-times. Many infants after waking from a morning or afternoon sleep are hungry but ill-humoured and crabby. Give a drink first and then follow this with a meal 20 to 30 minutes later or as soon as they are more awake and cheerful. 1–1¼ pints (575–700 ml) milk in total per day is sufficient, and greater quantities may diminish the appetite for other foods.

DON'T press foods at times they are not required. If toddlers are only hungry once a day make this the main meal and have well-spaced regular intervals when other food is offered, but do not make a child last so long between meals that he has gone past the point of no return and is too fatigued and exhausted to eat. A fairly regular routine is usually the most successful for children of this age regarding eating, exercise and sleeping to avoid tantrums, fatigue and frustration.

Improving the diet

Where a toddler's diet is not well balanced from choice seek one or more of the following solutions to ensure he remains in good health.

Diet Low in Vitamins A and D

Common imbalance when main foods consumed are chips, fish fingers, sausage, beans, crisps and biscuits.

1. Give correct dose of supplement as drops or pill of Vitamins A and D.
2. Give Cheddar type cheese and liver regularly.
3. Give carrots, dried apricots and yellow fruits for Vitamin A. Herring, sardine, or exposure to sunshine for Vitamin D.

Diet Low in Vitamin C

This occurs when fresh fruit and vegetables are not eaten and pop and squash replace fortified or real fruit juice.

1. Give Vitamin C fortified juice – rosehip, black-currant or orange – daily.
2. Give drops, powder or pill supplement of Vitamin C.
3. Serve tomato, green vegetables or fresh fruit three times daily.

Diet Low in B Vitamins

Common in small children with little appetite who take little meat, milk or eggs; also in children who over-eat or with high consumption of sugar or refined cereals where need is greater.

1. Choose breakfast cereals carefully and add wheatgerm. (See Chapter Six.)
2. Serve liver, kidney, yogurt, Marmite, wholemeal bread, peanut butter regularly.
3. Serve ¾–1 pint (425–575 ml) milk daily or add dried milk to foods.

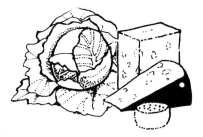

Diet Low in Calcium

Where milk and cheese are unpopular.

1. Encourage consumption of milk and variety of cheese, by 'disguising goodness' (see later in this chapter).
2. Use cottage cheese in desserts, fruit purées, and give custard and home-made ice creams.
3. Limit consumption of cocoa, chocolate, rhubarb, spinach and wholemeal flour which inhibit good absorption. Use carob powder for chocolate-type flavouring in drinks, etc.
4. Give Vitamin D supplement to aid absorption of calcium consumed.

Diet Low in Iron

Where eggs, meat and liver are unpopular.

1. Give plenty of Vitamin C for better absorption of iron.
2. Choose breakfast cereals reinforced with iron.
3. Serve liver once a week, use liver pâté in sand-wiches, add liver to mince, bolognese sauce and casseroles.
4. Most children remain very fit on well below recommended intake. Consult your doctor if you think your child anaemic. He will prescribe iron supplement if needed.

Diet Low in Protein

Where only pop, crisps and biscuits, sweets and ice cream are allowed to become a major part of the diet.

1. Replace crisps with nuts but do not leave child alone while eating them.
2. Give milk shakes with egg yolk plus extra dried milk added.
3. Make your own lollies and ice cream, adding plenty of dried and evaporated milk and eggs.
4. Give corned beef, chicken and cheese cut in fingers; they may be popular snacks.
5. Cut out completely all foods that contribute little to the diet. Hunger will make him eat other more suitable favourite foods, like fish fingers, beans, burgers, etc.

Will he starve?

You can be confident that he *won't*. Anorexia is a condition of adolescent girls largely, and there have only been a few rare cases of anorexia in small children who have been very seriously emotionally deprived. Your child can therefore be left to take as much food as he needs so far as calories are concerned and if thin this is probably his ideal weight.

Most people with faddy toddlers have children that are not underweight and are more often than not even quite chubby. Doctors and clinics will reassure you that your child is taking sufficient food as far as quantity is concerned. As far as quality is concerned, it will not be until such symptoms as anaemia appear that an inadequate diet is very obvious. Poor muscle tone, poor hair, nails, teeth, gums, easy bruising, dark rings around dull eyes and little resilience to infection will be other indications of poor diet. Poor physical growth with brittle bones and restricted intellectual development may take a long time to become obvious.

Many tests have been done on toddlers to see if they naturally choose food that they need. In spite of their strange idiosyncrasies – eating nothing but apples one day or cheese the next, going two to three days without a good meal then eating ravenously for several days on end – small children can largely be relied on to pick the food they need. *But*, to be more accurate, it was only those children tested who were offered *wholesome* alternatives – milk, fruit juices, meat, fish, eggs, cheese, cereal, bread, nuts, fruits and vegetables and food from simply prepared natural ingredients – who chose over a long period foods to meet all their nutritional requirements.

Today's children cannot be relied on to choose what they need if they have a free range of real food *and* all the commercial food products, sugar and sweets available. Only so long as their choice is restricted to foods which are of value can you be quite sure they will consume what their bodies need.

Do not worry if your child goes several days eating nothing but drinking milk or fruit juice (not pop or squash). Do not worry if he wants baked beans or fish fingers at every meal for a week. Don't worry if he smothers his food in ketchup (only those who drink half to one bottle per day have been known to suffer!). If he refuses vegetables offer more fruit; if he will not take milk, try yogurt or cheese. Over a period of time his fads and fancies will vary and overall, if only offered good food and no biscuits or other poor fillers, he will take a fairly balanced diet. Most minerals and some vitamins (not the B vitamins and Vitamin C, though) can be stored for several months so while a good daily intake is advisable it is not essential. A low intake of B vitamins tends to suppress appetite so ensure that foods rich in these are given as often as possible. Palatable preparations of the Vitamins A, D, and C are available and should be given daily.

Solving your toddler problems

Meal times can be very important to toddlers. If they wake at dawn, a drink of fruit juice or milk, or a bowl of cereal at the weekend, can be given to tide them over until a more civilised breakfast-time.

If time of lunch is geared to other members of the family or rest-times it will be necessary to decide if and when an elevenses will be served. A gap of three to four hours is reasonable for many between meals, but may be too big for some. Choose elevenses carefully depending on your child's appetite. If it is not good at lunch you may be giving an elevenses too high in calories. If milk and biscuits or sandwich are too much, switch to fruit juice and fruit.

It is wise to keep lunch at a regular time as children can become very difficult if they wait too long for meals and then are too bad-tempered or tired to eat.

Children and adults are healthier if they do not eat a big meal just before going to bed. Toddlers going to bed between 6 and 7 pm, therefore, should be given their last main meal of the day between 4 and 5 pm, with perhaps a milk drink as they go to bed. Foods are not well digested during sleep.

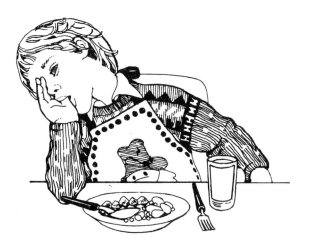

Energy from food is usually turned into fat deposits where it may stay, or it may just make your toddler awake and lively, refuelled with energy just when you want him to settle to sleep. Many who go to sleep on a full stomach have no interest in food at breakfast so if breakfast is not welcome check whether an evening meal is too late.

Refusing food

When children refuse food it is best to take a cheerful line even if you feel very annoyed having spent a lot of time and trouble preparing it. If refusal comes at a family meal leave food within the child's reach if he changes his mind and try and centre interest on something else – what you plan to do later that day. Avoid making an issue or scene; a relaxed comment like 'Oh, aren't you hungry' is quite enough comment; more persuasion is likely to lead to greater problems later. If there are tantrums see that the offender leaves the room and does not ruin the meal for others – but it usually takes two to make a tantrum! Avoid arguments, and don't cause a confrontation with remarks like 'If you don't eat this you can't have your pudding'. If a child refuses to eat and is clearly unwilling to join in the meal let him get down as soon as he wishes rather than allow him to become disruptive.

If you are on your own when a child refuses food try to sit down with him and have something to eat or drink yourself. It is a good idea if you can eat the same food or partly the same at lunch-time. Involve your toddler in some of the planning of meals – the shopping and preparation. Home-made beefburgers can be pressed into teddy-bear shaped cutters before cooking, and cheese on toast, toast, bread and sandwiches can be cut out with jolly cutters (they're called biscuit cutters but don't have to be used for biscuits). If well-meaning grannies, aunts or friends wish to give your child goodies try to steer them off sweets and ask for food cutters instead. Many can be bought singly or sets can be bought and distributed one at a time.

Try inviting his little friends to meals when he will be eating lunch or tea on his own. It will be good for both and it is amazing how the distraction will encourage him to eat with more relish. Try getting him up early enough to eat with the family if he does not eat breakfast cheerfully alone.

Make food more fun to eat. A small bowl of pâté or other dip can be given with a variety of items to dunk in – they love dunking toast in boiled eggs so make fingers of toast, carrot, cucumber, apple, pear etc. to dunk in a good nutritious dip.

Reluctant milk drinkers

By two or three years the ability to digest milk is substantially decreased in some people, who find it gives them indigestion. A reduction in the enzyme produced for digesting milk occurs in all, and in some may cause too large a curd developing when milk is in the stomach which is difficult for the body to digest. Some children find UHT (Long Life) or dried milks easier to digest, or boiled and cooled doorstep milk. Children should not be given skimmed milk constantly as it lacks Vitamins A and D. If you do have a problem with your child, try a variety of milks including goat's milk to see what suits. Persevere a little, and avoid adding chocolate or cocoa as some of the value of the milk will be lost. Carob, Horlicks or Ovaltine are more suitable flavourings, or add banana, stewed fruit, berries or currants or fruit yogurt to make a cold milk shake. Home-made yogurt drinks may also be more digestible for some. If all else fails try commercial milk shakes and flavoured milk but watch the sugar and chemical additive levels of your child's diet as a whole to ensure the total is comparatively low.

Dried milk can be discreetly added to mashed potato in quite large quantities for the reluctant drinker of milk. It may be added to soups, sauces, casseroles, crumble toppings or puddings. Evaporated milk can be used in home-made ice creams and lollies combined with fruit purées, as well as for mousses and jelly whips. Both these forms of milk are highly concentrated – 4½ heaped tablespoons dried and approximately half a large can evaporated milk equals 1 pint (575 ml). If only half of either of these can be added to a good diet daily, plus Vitamin D supplement, it will be a great help.

Cheese is an excellent alternative to milk; 1 oz (30 g) of a Cheddar type equals ¼ pint (150 ml) milk, but if this is also not liked, 1 oz (30 g) sardines and pilchards (with bone) are nutritionally as rich. Mash very finely in a blender or with a fork to make a pâté or paste, add tomato purée or lemon juice to make more palatable and use for sandwiches or combine with mashed potato (and dried milk) to make fish cakes for breakfast or tea. White fish is only a poor source of calcium so fish fingers are no substitute, I'm afraid.

Tea and coffee should *not* be given to young children. They both contain strong stimulants, both are high in caffeine, and recently coffee has been found to contain other addictive stimulants. Given with sugar added they are quickly preferred to plain milk which is then only taken reluctantly and often after considerable battles with the child.

Fun dips

Quick to make and highly nutritious, these are fun for a toddler to eat at lunch or tea.

BANANA, CHEESE AND PEANUT

½ banana
1–2 tablespoons low fat soft or cottage cheese
1 tablespoon smooth peanut butter

Purée through baby food mill or with potato masher. Use with apple, pear, cucumber, toast, fruit bread to dunk in or as sandwich filling.

TOMATO, CHEESE AND CHICKEN LIVER

¼ lb (115 g) chicken livers
1 tomato
1 tablespoon sunflower or corn oil
¼ lb (115 g) cream cheese

Thaw liver, fry quickly with halved tomato in hot oil until golden and just firm when pressed, about 3–4 minutes. Do not over-cook liver. Cool, and discard tomato skin. Purée with cheese. Freeze surplus for later. Use with carrot, cucumber, cauliflower, toast or bread or as a filling for jacket potato.

Nutritious soups

Serve in a mug or with bread to dunk in. Puréeing will disguise unpopular texture and make a nutritious soup for mother and toddler's lunch. Make for tea and use surplus in a thermos reheated next day for a packed lunch for Dad or older child.

LEEK AND POTATO SOUP

2 medium leeks
2 medium potatoes
1 tablespoon soft margarine
1½ pints (850 ml) milk
Salt and pepper
Dried milk powder (optional)

Wash and thickly slice leeks; peel and slice potatoes. Melt margarine in pan, add leeks and potatoes, cover and cook gently for 10–15 minutes without browning. Add milk and seasoning, cook for further 10–15 minutes until vegetables are soft. Purée finely, and add extra dried milk powder for any toddlers taking very little milk.

CAULIFLOWER SOUP

½ large or 1 small cauliflower
1 onion
½ pint (300 ml) water or stock
1 bay leaf
1 tablespoon margarine
1 tablespoon flour
1 pint (575 ml) milk
Salt, pepper and nutmeg
Dried milk powder (optional)

Chop cauliflower and onion. Cook in boiling water or stock until just tender, about 10–15 minutes, with bay leaf. Remove bay leaf, then purée finely. Melt margarine in pan, add flour and stir in milk and vegetable purée. Season with salt, pepper and nutmeg, bring to the boil. Add extra dried milk powder if needed. Float croûtons of grilled cheese on toast cut in dice on the soup or serve in fingers to dunk.

Disguising goodness

The following recipes are all for foods that are very popular with children. By adding *extra* and *good* ingredients, you can disguise the fact that you're increasing the nutritional values – and everyone will benefit!

BOLOGNESE SAUCE

½ lb (225 g) frozen chicken livers
½ lb (225 g) lean minced beef
1–2 cloves garlic (optional)
1 onion, sliced
3 sticks celery, sliced
1 medium tin tomatoes
1 teaspoon dried marjoram
Seasoning

Thaw livers in fridge for 24 hours. Fry mince slowly, stirring occasionally. Add liver, sliced garlic, onion and celery. Fry for 10 minutes until partly cooked. Add tomatoes, marjoram and seasoning. Simmer for 20 minutes. Purée sauce to a moderately smooth texture. Serve with cooked wholemeal pasta – small shapes, shells, wheels, etc. will be easier (and more fun) for a small child to eat than spaghetti. The sauce freezes well.

BEEF AND LIVER BURGERS

¼ lb (115 g) lamb or chicken liver
½ lb (225 g) lean minced beef
1 tablespoon grated onion
1 teaspoon mixed herbs
3 tablespoons soy sauce
1 small egg
½ teaspoon salt
4 tablespoons wholemeal breadcrumbs

Mince liver or purée in mixer or blender. Combine all ingredients, working together well. Shape with wet hands. Stack between layers of foil or kitchen film if freezing. Grill, fry or bake.

BRAN AND DATE LOAF

8 fl. oz (225 ml) milk
¼ lb (115 g) dates
1 egg
¼ lb (115 g) soft brown sugar
1 tablespoon Ovaltine or Horlicks
¼ lb (115 g) chopped mixed nuts or hazelnuts
¼ lb (115 g) All-Bran
3 teaspoons baking powder
6 oz (175 g) plain flour

Oven temperature: 180°C/350°F/Gas 4
2 lb (1 kg) loaf tin
Warm milk with dates, mash until soft and pulpy. Cool, adding egg, sugar, Ovaltine or Horlicks and nuts. Stir together well. When cold add All-Bran, sifted baking powder and flour, fold together and turn into tin. Bake 1 hour and test with fine skewer (if damp, the loaf isn't ready). Serve spread with cream cheese or peanut butter.

PEANUT AND MUESLI COOKIES

3 tablespoons soft margarine
2 tablespoons peanut butter (smooth or crunchy)
3 tablespoons soft brown sugar
4 tablespoons chopped raw peanuts
2 tablespoons milk
7 oz (200 g) muesli

Oven temperature: 190°C/375°F/Gas 5
7 × 11 inch (17.5 × 27.5 cm) biscuit tin, greased
Beat together margarine, peanut butter and sugar until well blended. Add nuts, milk and muesli. Stir together well and press into tin. Bake 10–15 minutes until golden. Mark into fingers. Leave to cool until tepid then lift onto wire rack to harden.

ROSEHIP AND APRICOT ICE CREAM

5 oz (150 g) dried apricots
⅓ pint (200 ml) boiling water
2 eggs
4 tablespoons rosehip syrup
1 small tin evaporated milk, chilled

Pour boiling water on apricots and leave to soak 24 hours. Simmer if not quite soft, then purée and chill. Separate eggs; whisk whites to a snow, then gradually whisk in apricot purée and rosehip syrup, keeping mixture firm. Lastly whisk in yolks. With clean whisk whip milk until thick. Fold in apricot/egg mixture and freeze.

HONEY AND APPLE FOOL

1 lb (450 g) apples
3 tablespoons water
1 tablespoon honey
6–8 tablespoons dried milk powder

Peel, slice and cook apples with water and honey. Cool and then purée with milk powder.

YOGURT LOLLIES

½ pint (300 ml) pure orange or pineapple juice
1 small carton plain yogurt
1 tablespoon thin honey
2 tablespoons dried milk powder

Use jar, tin or carton juice and combine all ingredients, whisking well, and turn into lolly or ice cube tray with lolly sticks. If blackcurrant, rosehip or concentrated sweetened orange juice are used, omit honey and use 3–4 tablespoons diluted with water.

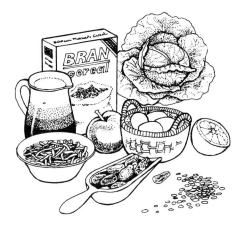

Comparison of some of previous recipes with commercial and other favoured foods

	Calories 1200–1400	Protein 25–40 g	Fat —	Carbohydrate —	Calcium 500 mg	Iron 7–8 mg	Vit. A 300 mcg	Vit. B₁ Thiamin 0.6 mg	Vit. B₂ Riboflavin 0.7 mg	Nicotinic Acid 8–9 mg	Vit. C 20 mg	Vit. D 10 mcg
Nutritional requirements 2–4 years	1200–1400	25–40 g	—	—	500 mg	7–8 mg	300 mcg	0.6 mg	0.7 mg	8–9 mg	20 mg	10 mcg
fish fingers 30 g (1 oz)	51	3.6	2.1	4.6	12.0	.2	0	.03	.03	.9	0	0
1 beef chipolata sausage	4	2.7	6.8	3.3	14.0	.4	.0	.01	.04	2.0	0	0
beef and liver burger 60 g (2 oz)	103	8.5	5.7	8.7	9.7	2.2	765	.07	.4	3.7	4.2	.19
bolognese sauce 100 g (3½ oz)	110	10.3	7.0	.3	16.6	3.4	437	.1	.8	6.0	12.0	.19
baked beans 100 g (3½ oz)	63	5.1	0.4	10.3	45.0	1.4	50	.07	.05	1.4	3.0	0
chips 100 g (3½ oz)	236	3.8	9.0	37.3	14.0	1.5	0	.01	.04	2.2	6.0	0
1 tablespoon roasted peanuts	146	12.0	18.0	2.1	15.0	.5	0	.6	.02	5.2	0	0
chocolate biscuit 30 g (1 oz)	141	2.0	7.7	18.5	37.0	.9	0	.03	.01	.5	0	0
1 medium slice white bread	125	4.0	.8	27	50	.8	0	.09	.01	1.3	0	0
1 medium slice wholemeal bread	120	4.7	1.5	23	24	1.5	0	.12	.04	1.0	0	0
vanilla ice cream 100 g (3½ oz)	192	4.1	11.3	19.8	137	.3	1	.05	.2	1.1	1	0
rosehip and apricot ice cream 60 g (2 oz)	106	6.1	3.7	13.5	68	.6	131	.2	.15	1.6	11.0	.75
milk 100 ml (3½ fl oz)	65	3.3	3.8	4.8	120	.1	44	.94	.15	.9	1.0	.05
1 egg	84	7.8	6.2	0	30	1.2	80	.04	.26	2.2	0	.8
Cheddar cheese 30 g (1 oz)	103	6.2	8.6	0	202	.15	105	.01	.12	1.3	0	.10
fruit yogurt 90 g (3 oz)	140	7.0	1.5	26.0	225	.5	15	.05	.35	1.5	0	0
yogurt lolly 90 g (3 oz)	90	3.7	2.3	14.4	122	.6	30	.08	.2	1.1	13.0	.9
honey and apple fool 90 g (3 oz)	120	4.7	4.3	16.5	151	1.3	57	.06	.24	1.2	12.0	2.0
1 banana	76	1.1	0	19.2	7	.4	33	.04	.07	.8	10.0	0
1 packet potato crisps	160	1.1	9.0	13.0	10	.5	0	.05	.02	1.8	0	0

Home from Playgroup Blues

Many three- to five-year-olds return home from playgroup or school too exhausted or excited to face a large meal. They need refuelling but may have a greater need for a sleep or a period of relaxation before facing a proper meal. If your youngster clearly needs food but is not in the right frame of mind to settle happily to a meal it may be better to give an appealing snack or nourishing drink to get him through this difficult period, giving nourishment and a few calories without spoiling his appetite for a proper meal later. Sweets, biscuits, chips and chocolate will all dampen the appetite and provide little in the way of nourishment. When the daily intake of food is small as it invariably is for younger children, it is important that *all* food given is nutritious. Small items on sticks or to eat in fingers may be more tempting than tackling a meal with knife and fork for a tired child. A good nutritious *drink* may be the answer, and extra-wide straws are available for milk shakes and will make them more popular. Or he may appreciate a mug of soup.

COLD KEBABS

Chunks of meat, sausage, ham, spam, chicken or cheese with pieces of apple, banana, pineapple, melon, grapes (seeded), peach, pear, apricot, tangerine, orange, cucumber, radish, raw mushroom, carrot, celery, tomato. Use cocktail sticks if wished.

BACON AND KIDNEY ROLY POLY

Half rasher bacon wrapped round quarter or half kidney. Bake or grill until golden. Small chunks of liver may replace kidney.

KIDNEY AND TOMATO SOUP

1/2 lb (225 g) ox kidney
1 level tablespoon flour
1 tablespoon soft margarine
1 onion, sliced
1 pint (575 ml) chicken stock or vegetable water
15 oz (425 g) tin tomatoes
Seasoning
1/2 teaspoon rosemary or thyme

Cut core from kidney and thickly slice. Dust with flour and fry briskly in fat with onion until brown. Add stock or vegetable cooking water, plus tin of tomatoes, seasoning and herbs. Simmer gently for 30–40 minutes until kidney is tender. Purée soup finely. Freeze if wished.

BANANA EGG NOG

1/3 pint (200 ml) milk
1 tablespoon dried milk powder
1/2 egg or 1 yolk
1/2–1 small banana
1 tablespoon rosehip or orange juice

Heat milk if preferred warm. Place all ingredients in an electric blender. Purée to a frothy texture. A tablespoon of wheatgerm may be added for those who like a rougher texture.

BLACKCURRANT MILK SHAKE

1/3 pint (200 ml) milk
2–3 tablespoons cottage cheese
1 tablespoon blackcurrant syrup

Place in electric blender and purée to a good velvety froth.

LEMON AND HONEY NOG

1 large lemon
1/2 egg or 1 yolk
1 small carton plain yogurt
1 'carton' milk
2–3 teaspoons honey

Grate rind and squeeze juice of lemon. Use yogurt carton to measure milk. Mix all together in an electric blender.

APRICOT MILK SHAKE

1/3 pint (200 ml) milk
4 tablespoons apricot purée
1 tablespoon orange or lemon juice

Make apricot purée with fresh, dried or frozen fruit or use tinned apricots in fruit juice. Freeze purée in ice cube trays and thaw 3–4 cubes to add to milk shake. Purée drink in blender.

Toddlers in the kitchen

The kitchen is a room to which the whole family gravitates. As mother, you spend a large part of the day here and small children will want to be with you constantly. But hot pans, irons, toasters and water make it a potentially hazardous room, so your activities and the positions of equipment need planning to avoid many dangers.

1. Do not leave small children in the kitchen when you go to the door, telephone, bathroom. Always take your toddler out and shut the door.

2. Check all flexes of kettle, toaster, mixers, etc. Fold up surplus length and secure with tape or rubber bands so not left dangling. Take care never to leave the iron to cool or heat up unattended with flex dangling. A rack fixed to the wall or a high, tiled shelf or window-sill are good positions. Make sure you have sufficient power points in safe places.

3. Avoid deep-fat frying if possible; it is the greatest source of danger in the kitchen. When you are distracted by the urgent demands of a toddler (calling for the potty, for instance) you are not likely to be as reliable in your concentration. Use oven chips (if you must serve chips) and oven-bake or grill instead of frying.

4. Check your cooker. The heat of the exterior of many oven doors (and Agas) reach temperatures high enough to cause second-degree burns. British standards allow temperatures up to 120°C (248°F) on the outside of the door, far hotter than boiling water. Those with glass centre panels become very hot. Some cookers only reach 40–50°C (104–122°F) but even this will feel very hot to a toddler. When infants first get on their feet to walk round furniture, they are at great risk of burns from oven doors and central heating radiators: they will not be steady enough to jump back quickly and can stay leaning on the burning surface in terror. Check your oven door after the oven has been on very high temperature for 15 to 20 minutes.

5. Check tops of cookers; knobs should be child-proof or out of reach. Use back burners in preference to front. Leave pan handles turned backwards or inwards but be careful these do not get too hot when you handle them.

6. Plan your kitchen so that pans or kettles of boiling water are not carried across the room. With toddlers around and toys on the floor, this is very hazardous.

7. Check contents of all low cupboards in the kitchen to ensure they are safe. Use for pans, plastic or metal cooking ware, baking tins, tinned goods, cereals – items that are unbreakable and safe.

8. Store very safely all cleaning chemicals, bleach, detergent, aerosol cans, oven cleaners, etc., as well as vitamin supplements and aspirin that you might keep in the kitchen. A high or locked cupboard is best.

9. Use a safety gate with your child and his toys just outside the kitchen if at all possible, particularly if the kitchen is small. If your kitchen is large, use a playpen for as long as possible.

Kitchen Creations

Children can learn through 'cooking', and allowing them to take part will stimulate their interest in food and the fun of preparing it – even at this early stage.

PRINTING

Some root vegetables can be cut to make interesting shapes for printing. You can carve out decorations for your child using potatoes, carrots, swede, etc. Dip in ink or brush with paint and press down on fabric, paper, ribbon, etc. Other items will make interesting textures without carving, such as halved onion, sprout, lemon, apple.

MULTI-COLOUR WAX CRAYONS

Place old bits of crayons with a bit of candle in small tin-foil containers. Bake in hot oven (200°C/400°F/ Gas 6) for a few minutes until melted. Leave to cool without stirring for new fun crayons.

SPROUTING SEEDS

Mustard and cress was for years the favourite, grown on blotting paper, old flannel, sand-filled yogurt pots, egg cartons, even egg shells. It will take about seven days until the results are ready for cropping in a warm kitchen.

Bean sprouts, using green mung beans or alfalfa, take about four days to germinate. Many of the dried peas and beans are excellent to grow and fun to eat – black-eyed beans, whole lentils, and peas. Red kidney beans are the only variety not recommended: when well sprouted they are said not to be toxic but since they are toxic normally before proper cooking it is best if they are sprouted to use in cooked dishes, not salads.

Buy seeds for sprouting from grocers and health-food shops, not seed merchants where they will be more expensive. Sprouted seeds are very rich nutritionally and develop more vitamins than the food from which they were sprouted.

Place a couple of tablespoons of seeds in a large empty jar. Add tepid water, cover with a piece of J-cloth and secure with rubber band. Tip off water leaving contents wet. Rinse beans with warm water morning and evening for four days or until well sprouted. Store in very warm dark place. When grown keep beans in fridge and use within two to three days in salad sandwiches and stir-fry vegetables.

PASTRY MAKING

Always a popular pastime with toddlers. Use your own home-made or frozen pastry. Let children roll out and wrap round quartered cored apples, pears, stoned plums, apricots, pieces of rhubarb, whole gooseberries or spoonful of other berries and currants – all better than endless jam tarts. Try savoury tart fillings of leftover chopped vegetables with grated cheese, spoonfuls of baked beans, savoury mince or fish mixture; chopped meat, ham or bacon, and beaten egg.

GINGERBREAD MEN

½ teaspoon ginger
½ teaspoon bicarbonate of soda
4 heaped tablespoons plain flour
2 heaped tablespoons soft brown sugar
1 heaped tablespoon soft margarine
1 heaped tablespoon golden syrup

Oven temperature: 160°C/325°F/Gas 3

Place in bowl in order given to save washing spoon! Stir together to a firm paste. Model or cut into gingerbread men, then decorate with currants for buttons and sliced glacé cherries for eyes and mouth if wished. Bake until golden, and cool until tepid on baking tray. Lift off with fish slice.

FINGER PAINTING

½ cup cornflour
2 tablespoons sugar
2 cups water
1 teaspoon washing-up liquid
Food colouring

Mix cornflour and sugar with a little water to a smooth paste, add remainder of water, bring to boil stirring constantly and cook ½–1 minute. Add washing-up liquid for easy cleaning later, divide between three to five pots and add colour to each. Children can use fingers, cotton-wool buds, paint or pastry brushes. Do not store.

Aerosol shaving cream may also be coloured for finger paints.

NO-COOK PLAYDOUGH

Supply a little rolling pin (short length of thick dowelling or broom handle), biscuit cutters, bottle tops and egg cups as cutters, as well as dried beans, peas and pasta shapes for extra creativity. It is cheaper than plasticine, edible if they want to eat it, and is very easy to vacuum off the carpet!

1 cup flour
1 cup salt
2 tablespoons vegetable oil
Food colouring
1 teaspoon alum or glycerine (optional)
⅓–½ cup water

Work the ingredients together, adding water gradually until like a bread dough. This can be done best in a mixer. Alum or glycerine retard drying. Store separate colours in plastic bags when not in use, preferably in the fridge.

Bake shaped dough in cool oven for several hours (like meringues) to keep for posterity if wished! Paint with water colours or poster or acrylic paints. Glaze with varnish or nail polish. Excellent for ornaments, pendants or key-ring decorations, as Christmas presents or decorations. Press in small piece of cut drinking straw to make a hole for hanging.

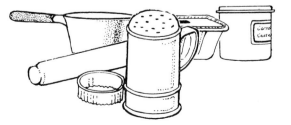

Chapter Six
The over-fives

The period between five and eleven years is the one in which you can most influence your childrens' eating habits and the patterns they will develop for life. If you have fed them wisely over the years, and continue to do so, it is these good eating routines of home that they will consider the norm, and will take with them into their lives outside the home. For this is also the time that they start school, when you will have less and less control of what they eat – at school lunch, for instance – or how they spend their pocket money. In order for them to choose wisely, they need to have a basic understanding of nutrition instilled into them in these important years, *before* they reach eleven.

By five, children are largely past the early fussier stage; their natural appetite is increasing and most enjoy food. By seven, they will be increasingly taking the responsibility of choosing food for themselves, and by eleven, at secondary school stage, they are likely to have a considerable choice in one of the main meals of the day. About one-third of their daily intake of nutrients and calories may be taken at lunch-time, and with modern canteen-style self-service, and relatively unlimited use of fish and chip shops, this can result in an appalling choice of diet – just chips, buns, sweets and pop.

Nutrition as a subject is rarely taught in school before secondary school age, and children's information before eleven comes from their homes, and largely from television commercials. Do point out to children, from an early age and regularly, the purpose of television food advertising. It is to sell more of a manufacturer's product to make bigger profits; it is not designed to tell people what they *need* to eat (except perhaps the Milk Marketing Board commercials). Jingles like 'A chocolate bar a day helps you work, rest and play' should be rewritten by the family as 'A chocolate bar a day helps your teeth rot away' – which is much nearer the truth. Encourage your children to reword other advertising jingles similarly, so that they do not absorb them unthinkingly, but view them more objectively.

Encourage them also to read the list of contents on packaged or tinned food, and point out the undesirable chemical colours, flavours and other additives which they may contain. When shopping with them, teach them by example how to choose wisely: checking prices; selecting fruit and vegetables for quality and nutritional value; by buying the meat with the lowest fat content; and by reading the contents or ingredients on processed foods, burgers, sausages, tinned and packet foods. They will quickly learn to be selective instead of idly clamouring for rubbishy junk foods (and incidentally will have unnoticed lessons in mathematics, biology and reading!).

Ultimately your children will need to learn to cook and this is as important for boys as girls. A major part of growing up and independence for both sexes is the ability to look after themselves adequately. Teenagers can be notoriously uncooperative, so 'teaching' them at home before they reach this stage, is by far the best idea. School cookery for the secondary school-age is still largely based on the art of pastry- and cake-making (of little value in a proper diet), so let them 'help' and develop an interest in food and cookery from as early an age as possible.

Meal planning

The times of meals can affect not only your child's enjoyment of food but also his body's ability to use nutrients well.

Most children under eleven should aim to have their last main meal of the day between 4 and 5 o'clock. This is particularly important for younger children. If food is eaten as early as this, it will provide a burst of energy as a result of refuelling.

Children should then have the opportunity to use this energy in lively activity, so that by 6 to 7 pm the younger children will then be able to relax and should readily sleep. If young children simply sit watching TV for some hours, then the burst of energy will come at 8 or 9 pm, just when you want them to sleep. Older children of nine to eleven years may be able to wait until about 6 pm for their meal, but should not be encouraged to last until as late as 7, otherwise they will not have time to digest their food before going to bed.

The practice of giving a milk drink at bedtime is helpful for many since milk is easy to digest, but this should not be accompanied by other food. During the night the digestive system should be given a rest so that the child sleeps more soundly, and there is as little stress on all the organs of the body as possible. The heart, for example, has to work harder to pump blood round the digestive system if a large meal is eaten before going to bed, and food not properly digested may cause a feeling of nausea in the morning when more should be taken. It is unlikely that a child who last had a good meal at 4 pm will not be really quite hungry at breakfast, which should be the most important meal of the day.

Surplus nutrients from one day's food are not always carried over to the next. B vitamins and Vitamin C will be excreted and protein converted to fat. Toxic wastes will be produced as a result of the breakdown of foods into basic nutrients. If the nutrients are not replaced and the body wastes in the bowel and urine are not excreted there will be a greater tendency towards headaches, crabbiness, and poor concentration during the morning. Foods taken at breakfast should have plenty of fibre and fluid to help eliminate waste products, and should provide protein, B vitamins, Vitamin C and energy for a good start to the day.

One-quarter of the population of the UK eat no breakfast. This must represent a vast amount of inefficiency and bad temper, so every effort should be made to train children in the habit of eating breakfast. This will be partly achieved by good example and partly by the times of meals and activity of the previous evening. Those children or adults who take quite a time to fully wake in the morning should be woken early enough (so should go to bed early enough) to have sufficient time to play and get dressed before having breakfast, so that there is a greater chance of them being in the mood to eat.

Girls, particularly as they approach their teens, need to have meal-times and sleeping habits carefully watched since they are the most likely to give up eating breakfasts. Make sure that bed-time snacks are rigidly controlled for those who are reluctant to eat breakfast. Some children can cope with a tea plus quite a substantial snack later in the evening, yet still eat a hearty breakfast. Those children can obviously be safely left to follow their own natural inclinations if their weight is normal.

A further advantage in not eating food later in the day is that the energy value in the meals eaten before 5 pm is likely to be completely burned up and not converted to fat deposits. Food which is given little opportunity of being burned up in activity sports – bicycling, active play, or for adults jogging, squash, etc. – is likely to be converted to fat deposits and may lead to a greater tendency to overweight. This is a particularly useful argument for older girls.

Between-meal snacks

Break-time snacks for most who eat a good breakfast can be very small. A drink of milk, fruit drink or squash is suitable. For those who are hungry, a few nuts or raisins or a piece of fruit are a better choice than biscuits. An apple is the most portable, least crushable or messy, so it is the ideal choice to stuff in a satchel or pocket for school.

Dentists come out firmly in favour of crisps etc. instead of sweets or biscuits as a snack as they are less likely to set up tooth decay. But before you make this choice it is worth remembering that all these are very high in salt. The habit of eating very salty foods

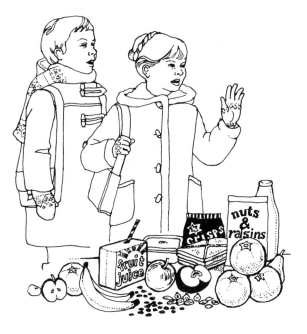

makes the palate less sensitive to salt so more is often liberally sprinkled on other foods at meal-times to make them seem less bland. In the short term, this excess salt means loss of potassium, thus muscular fatigue, but in the long term, although it's difficult to seriously consider when your child is only five years old, you might be pointing him towards premature heart disease, high blood pressure and strokes. It is sadly true that these diseases are already hitting a much larger number of young people between thirty and forty-five. A high salt intake is a major contributory factor, and young children are now eating a very much higher quantity of these salty foods than ten to twenty years ago.

Children who eat a poor breakfast, or only a small bowl of cereal, may need a sandwich with a protein filling at break-time to tide them over until lunch. Do not give too much, which might take the edge off the lunch-time appetite. Pack in a small plastic box so that it is not mangled by break-time.

After school many children are quite weary. The sooner they are fed the better, but if very young children are too tired to face a whole meal when they get home, give a drink of milk and follow the ideas for tired children home from playgroups in the previous chapter.

Food chosen for tea-time should balance the meals earlier in the day so that the whole intake provides the child's nutritional requirements for his age. It is tempting to give a drink and biscuit when a child gets home from school and then make him wait for a late family meal. This is not in his best interests if he is only five to seven years old and if the family meal is after 6.30. When older children would like to join in a family meal at this time it may be a good idea to give them one course of their meal at 4 pm, and let them join in the dessert at the family meal later, so they do not consume too much at this time and spoil their night's sleep or chance of a good breakfast.

Pocket money and sweets

Pocket money presents a thorny problem in relation to food. Before giving pocket money regularly, it is important to work out how you think it might be spent and how you think it should be spent. If you expect it all to be spent on sweets, investigate their current cost, how many sweets you think he should be allowed to eat, then base your allowance on this. If you do not wish him to use this money on sweets it will need to be made clear from the start. If you expect money to be split between sweets, toys and

comics etc., it may be wise to have clear rules concerning this, or give out the money on separate occasions for children under seven to eight years, to ensure that all of it is not spent on unsuitable food. Handling and managing money is a natural part of a child's education and, although it may create difficulties, it is important that children learn the value of money and how to purchase wisely.

Breakfasts

Breakfast is the most important meal of the day, particularly for children. It gives every one the energy and vitality to start the day, and for children of between three and eleven, this means coping with a morning at school or playgroup. School timetables for those under twelve are worked out on the assumption that childrens' concentration is at its peak in the morning, and lessons in the 3 Rs are concentrated at this time. In the afternoon the concentration is presumed to be diminished, so less difficult subjects like art, music, sports, games and play activities are planned for much of that session.

Children who eat little or no breakfast have been found to have a considerably poorer performance at school in the first half of the day and only achieve their potential after they have eaten lunch. Their educational attainments in reading, writing and number work obviously suffer most.

The choice of food at breakfast should be based on the body's most urgent needs. Calories will be needed for energy; fibre and fluid to stimulate the working of the digestive system to eliminate quickly the toxic wastes of the previous day. This will promote a feeling of well-being as will the intake of B vitamins, Vitamin C and protein.

Breakfast should therefore concentrate on the supply of the following nutrients.
Protein: Milk, cereal, bread, egg, bacon, baked beans etc.
B Vitamins: Milk, reinforced cereals, egg, baked beans, bread, bacon etc.
Vitamin C: Fresh fruit, tomatoes, fruit juices or supplement.
Fibre: High and moderately high fibre cereals, baked beans, whole fruit.
Fluid: Milk, fruit juice, weak milky tea and weak coffee (only for children over seven).
Energy: Carbohydrate, milk, cereals, bread, baked beans, fats in butter or margarine, egg, sausage, bacon etc.

Reluctant breakfast eaters

Many people are 'day birds', who wake bright and breezy, happily munch through a good breakfast and make good use of their time at the beginning of the day. Most will need no encouragement to eat breakfast as they are genuinely hungry; they will enjoy a bowl of cereal and are happy to eat a cooked breakfast or anything else in sight. But many are 'night owls', who are reluctant to go to sleep at night, and in a bad humour in the morning. They do not feel like eating breakfast and the thought of food makes them feel awful. It is most important that this natural tendency is not allowed to hamper their school attainment, even their whole future, and the answer to this problem probably lies in the eating pattern of the previous day. (See *Meal Planning* for over-fives).

Tempt reluctant breakfast eaters with less conventional or *different* breakfasts. If they don't fancy cereals (and sweetened varieties can dampen the appetite), the digestive juices can be stimulated much more by savoury foods or even fresh fruit. They may enjoy breakfast much more if they start with a few mouthfuls of cheese, bacon, sausage, fish fingers or baked beans, scrambled egg or herb omelette, or even toast and Marmite which will stimulate the flow of saliva. The conventional giving of cereal first is merely so that the cook can get on with making toast and other foods. Or you can try some of the ideas in the following recipes. *Any* effort is worthwhile if your reluctant breakfast eater eventually does have a better breakfast and so improves his academic chances.

But if all else fails and juggling the time of evening meals does not seem to be the answer, the breakfast-less child should go off to school (or work if it is Dad or older child), taking with them a suitable snack to eat at the earliest possible time.

Break-time milk is a perfect snack but it is possible that your child may be interested in food even earlier. Sticky buns, biscuits and crisps are a very poor snack with which to start the day. The food should provide as many of the nutrients of a good breakfast as possible. Send with:

● A carton or mug of milk or fruit juice plus cheese or hard-boiled egg and crackers or plain wholemeal biscuits.

● Sandwich filled with peanut butter, egg, cheese, liver pâté or meat filling.

● Pot of yogurt.

● Tea cake with cottage or curd cheese, or peanut butter.

● Fruit, fresh or dried.

● Muesli biscuit.

These snacks can be eaten at break-time or, better still, on the way to school or before school in the playground. The sooner your child eats, the better will be his performance at morning school.

Breakfast cereals

Of the wide range of breakfast cereals available the nutritional value and price per ounce is very revealing. When they are compared as in the chart following, it is surprising to see how some contribute so much less nutritionally yet are comparatively expensive – Rice Krispies, for instance. And the bulk of some makes it difficult to assess the real value and cost.

The caloric value of most cereals is very similar per ounce but the protein value varies considerably as do the minerals and vitamins. Most have valuable reinforcements of iron and B vitamins; only a few have calcium. It should be remembered that supplements of Vitamins A and D are toxic if taken in too great a quantity; those taking Readybrek and Grape-Nuts should not take additional supplements of the above vitamins as drops or tablets every day as a 1 oz (30 g) quantity of these cereals will supply much of their needs. Vitamin reinforcements of different brands of cornflakes etc., do vary a little; Vitamins B_6, and B_{12} and folic acid are not added to all. Choose those with the best supplements.

Very high bran cereals like All-Bran and Farm-house Bran are not suitable for small children. These should only be used if constipation is a problem and then used only as much, or as long, as is necessary. Too high a level of bran in the diet of small children will limit the absorption of minerals and vitamins from their food. Cornflakes, Rice Krispies and other cereals with a very low fibre content should be served with a high bran cereal on alternate days or combined, unless wholemeal bread and plenty of bran in other foods is supplied.

Ensure that children who eat breakfast cereal and no cooked breakfast choose the cereal with the highest possible protein content – ProNutro or Readybrek – with plenty of milk. A few Frosties, Coco-Pops or Ricicles are a poor start to the day on their own.

Hot cereals

Most cereals do not take long to cook, and it is not only oats that can be made into a delicious hot breakfast cereal.

Add cereals to cold water or milk, or a mixture of

Guide to making a good choice of cereals

Per 30g (1oz)	Calories K Cal	Protein grams	Fat grams	Carbo. grams	Fibre grams	Calc. mg	Iron mg	Vit A mcg	Thi. B$_1$ mg	Ribo. B$_2$ mg	Pyri. B$_6$ mg	Folic Acid mg	Nico. Acid mg
Bran Flakes	85	2.8	.3	19	4.0	0	11.4	0	.28	.43	.51	0	4.6
Readybrek	106	4.0	2.2	18	2.1	34	5.7	342	.5	.65	0	0	7.7
Oats	113	3.4	2.5	20.6	2.7	16	1.2	0	.14	.03	NA	0	.8
Oatgerm and Bran	109	4.3	.9	16.9	4.86	NA	4.1	0	1.1	.05	.1	NA	NA
Wheatflakes	96	3.0	.6	19.0	3.0	NA	1.7	0	.2	.28	NA	NA	2.85
Weetabix	87	3.0	.6	17.2	3.5	NA	1.7	0	NA	.28	NA	NA	2.85
Cornflakes (fortified)	100	2.2	.2	24.2	1.4	1	.1	0	.32	.4	.5	.86	3.0
All-Bran	71	4.0	0	12.7	8.1	0	2.5	0	.28	.43	.5	NA	4.6
Home-made muesli	77.5	2.2	2.4	12.6	3.0	34	.6	20	.06	.04	NA	NA	.5
Shreddies	Similar to Weetabix – no iron												
Rice Krispies	100	1.7	0	NA	1.4	0	1.9	0	.28	.43	.5	0	2.85
Grape Nuts	104	2.5	NA	NA	NA	NA	NA	380	.37	.43	.5	.114	5
Coco-Pops/Frosties/ Ricicles	100	1.4	0	NA	1.4	0	1.9	0	.28	.43	.5	0	2.85
Crunchy Nut Flakes	107	2.2	NA	NA	1.4	0	1.9	0	.28	.43	.5	0	2.85
Special K	100	5.4	.1	20	1.4	1	3.8	0	.34	.48	16	0	5.2
Baby's mixed cereal	112	4.6	1.3	20	low	200	5.7	22.8	.14	.2	.3	.02	3.1
2 tsp sugar	56	0	0	15.0	0	0	0	0	0	0	0	0	0
100 ml (3½ fl. oz) milk	65	3.3	3.8	4.8	0	120	.1	44	.04	.15	.04	.05	.9
Wheatgerm	85	7.0	NA	10.0	NA	NA	2.5	0	.4	.16	.23	NA	1.5

Key

Carbo.	Carbohydrate.
Calc.	Calcium.
Thi.	Thiamin.
Ribo.	Riboflavin.
Pyri.	Pyridoxine.
Nico.	Nicotinic.
NA	Figures not available.

● The bulk of many cereals makes price comparison difficult at first glance. However, most cereals provide about 100 calories per 30 g (1 oz) and this is a realistic serving. Nutritional composition lists on packets are usually given for 100 g (3½ oz) (eg 6 Weetabix) which gives a misleading impression – small children may only take 15 g (½ oz).

● Bought and home-made muesli usually contain 2–3 g fibre, occasionally up to 5. Their nutritional value is otherwise similar to oats. Nuts and dried fruits increase value. Prices range from 3–7p. These cereals are not usually fortified with additional vitamins or minerals. If grains are unheated in the processing they will contain many valuable trace vitamins not listed here.

● Many ready-sweetened cereals can be more than 50% sugar. *Do* be critical and taste all you give to your children.

B$_{12}$	C	D	E	Approx. price per 30 g (1 oz) in mid 1983	
mcg	mg	mcg	mg		
0	10	3.6	0	4p	**Bran Flakes**
0	11	4.9	0	3½p	**Readybrek**
0	0	0	NA	2p	**Oats**
0	0	0	1.0	4p	**Oatgerm and Bran**
NA	0	0	0	2p	**Wheatflakes**
NA	0	0	0	3p	**Weetabix**
.5	0	0	0	3p	**Cornflakes (fortified)**
NA	0	.8	NA	2½p	**All-Bran**
NA	1.5	.3	NA	4p	**Home-made muesli**
					Shreddies
.5	0	.8	0	5½p	**Rice Krispies**
1.4	0	1.0	0	4p	**Grape Nuts**
0	0	0	0	5–5½p	**Coco-Pops/Frosties/Ricicles**
0	0	0	0	6p	**Crunchy Nut Flakes**
0	0	.3	0	7p	**Special K**
.08	14.3	.26	NA	7p	**Baby's mixed cereal**
0	0	0			**2 tsp sugar**
.3	2.0	2.91	.09		**100 ml (3½ fl. oz) milk**
0	0	0	3.1	6p	**Wheatgerm**

● The tiny cereal packets in sets of 6 contain about 15 g (½ oz) each, 90 g (3 oz) in total and represent very poor value for money, about 19p per 30 g (1 oz)!

● All-Bran is not suitable for small children. It is too high in fibre.

● Own-brand supermarket products may have a lower level of added vitamins etc. Check when comparing prices.

● Specially designed baby cereals are the most suitable under one year but may be gradually replaced by ProNutro and Readybrek or occasionally Weetabix between ten to fifteen months.

Cooking Cereals

1 Cup Uncooked cereal	Cups of Liquid	Cooking Time (minutes)
Oatmeal	2½	5
Rolled and jumbo oats	3	35–45
Cornmeal/maize	4–6	10
Wholewheat	2–4	5
Cracked wheat	2	15
Buckwheat	2	20
Semolina	2	5
Rye flour	3	20
Rolled rye (flakes)	2	5
Millet	2	30
Brown rice	2	45
Ground brown rice	4–6	15
Hominy	3	2 hours

both, and stir occasionally as they come to the boil, or sprinkle on to boiling liquid, stirring just enough to prevent lumps. Do not over-stir or cereals will become gluey. They may have extra dried milk stirred in before serving for a creamy texture. Many are excellent cooked slowly in slow cookers or at the bottom of an Aga or solid-fuel cooker overnight.

Extra interest can be added by tossing in dried fruits, chopped nuts, coconut or topped with spoonfuls of cottage cheese or yogurt. For a chocolate flavour add carob powder. For other flavours try cinnamon, nutmeg, cloves, peanut butter, honey, fruit purée, fruit juice, raspberries, blackberries, strawberries etc.

Cereals may be cooked in quantity and stored, unflavoured, in the refrigerator for re-heating for up to seven days. Cover well to prevent skin forming when storing or cooling. Many find cereal tastes better and is more easily digested on re-heating. Small quantities left over can be stirred into casseroles and stews to thicken them or added to soups.

Since extra vitamins and iron are not added to home-cooked cereals they do not have such a high mineral and B vitamin content as the commercial cereals. They are, however, much cheaper and can be reinforced with milk powder and nutritious ingredients to make them more interesting. Those having a good cooked breakfast will find them more than adequate nutritionally.

Cooked breakfast

There is rather more to cooked breakfast than sausage, bacon and eggs. Try some of the following recipes, and I think even the most reluctant breakfast eater will change his mind!

EGGY BREAD

1 egg
4 tablespoons milk
1 tablespoon wheatgerm
2 slices bread

Beat egg, milk and wheatgerm together. Soak both sides of bread in the mixture and then fry on both sides in some sunflower oil or margarine.

BREAKFAST DROP SCONES

2 eggs
4 tablespoons self-raising flour
4 tablespoons milk
Seasoning

Separate yolks from whites, and whip whites until stiff. Whisk yolks, flour, milk and seasoning to a thick batter and fold together with whites. Drop spoonfuls into a hot frying pan with a little oil, and turn when golden.

Add any of the following variations to the batter if you like:
- 2–3 tablespoons chopped cooked bacon, chicken, ham, fish, liver, kidney or hard-boiled egg.
- 2–3 tablespoons grated Cheddar cheese.
- 1–3 tablespoons chopped herbs, nuts, apple or banana.

BREAKFAST KEDGEREE

¼ lb (115 g) cooked white or brown rice
2 teaspoons sunflower or corn oil
1 egg
2–5 oz (60–150 g) of one or more of:
white fish, smoked fish, hard-boiled egg, cheese, ham, bacon, kidney, liver, tomatoes, mushrooms

Cook rice the day before. Foil-wrap fish and bake in oven. Fry other chosen items in oil (bacon, kidney, liver, tomato or mushroom). When lightly cooked add rice, seasoning, herbs if wished, cooked chopped items and beaten raw egg. Heat gently stirring until all is hot but egg still creamy.

GRILLED CHEESY TOMATOES

Combine 1–2 tablespoons cottage cheese with some grated Cheddar. Grill halved tomatoes, skin side up. Turn over, set on bread slices, top with cheese mixture, and grill until bubbling.

BREAKFAST PIZZA

Use large scones, split baps, crumpets or slices of bread as base. Top with a sliced tomato or a tomato sauce, then add sardines, sliced ham, or just cheese and grill or bake until hot.

COTTAGE CHEESE AND FRUIT SALAD

Combine cottage cheese with chopped fruit or dried fruits and nuts.

BREAKFAST CAKES

Use equal quantities of mashed potato, and one of the protein ingredients from Column 1. Drop large spoonfuls into a coating from Column 2 and shape. Chill overnight and bake, fry or grill (cover wire grill with foil to prevent sticking) next day.

Column 1	*Column 2*
Cooked fresh fish	*Oatmeal*
Tinned fish	*Rolled oats*
Cooked kipper or smoked fish	*Jumbo oats*
Cooked kidney or liver	*White breadcrumbs*
Sausagemeat	*Wholemeal breadcrumbs*
Cooked chopped bacon, ham or chicken	*Rice Krispies, crushed*
Cooked chopped liver or liver pâté	*Wheatflakes*
Cottage or Cheddar cheese	*Grapenuts*
Cooked minced beef, lamb or pork	*Cracked wheat*
Cooked cabbage or sprouts	*Chopped nuts*
Cooked beans or lentils	*Flour*
Chopped hard-boiled eggs	*Rye flakes*

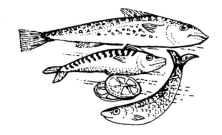

Unconventional breakfasts

These, too, should stir the imaginations of any reluctant to eat in the morning, and they make a delicious change even for those conventionally dedicated to bacon and eggs.

ORANGE AND BANANA BREAKFAST JELLY

generous ¾ pint (500 ml) carton or tinned orange juice
1 sachet gelatine
1–2 bananas

Make the jelly the day before. Soak gelatine in 4 tablespoons juice in small pan, and warm gently until crystals dissolve. Remove from heat, add remaining juice and sliced banana. Pour into three or four pots or cartons, and chill to set.

PEANUT CUSTARD

4 tablespoons hot milk
1 tablespoon peanut butter
1 egg

Pour hot milk on to peanut butter and mash until smooth. Beat in egg. Pour into small cup or pot, cover, and place in covered pan with just enough water to come half way up the side. Simmer for 7–12 minutes or until set.

BREAKFAST BISCUITS

4 oz (115 g) soft margarine
2 oz (60 g) brown sugar
1 large tablespoon runny honey
4 eggs
8 oz (225 g) wholemeal flour
4 tablespoons wheatgerm
4 oz (115 g) oatmeal
2 teaspoons baking powder
7 oz (200 g) raisins
4 oz (115 g) chopped or ground nuts

Oven temperature: 180°C/350°F/Gas 4

Beat together margarine, sugar, honey and eggs. Mix dry ingredients together so that baking powder is well distributed and fold all ingredients together. Turn into well greased small roasting tin. Bake for 30 minutes. Cut into squares while still warm.

TAHINI TOAST

1 tablespoon soya flour
1 tablespoon sesame seed paste (tahini)
3–4 tablespoons water
½ teaspoon honey
1–2 slices bread

Beat together soya flour, *tahini*, water and honey. Soak bread slices in mixture and fry on both sides in a little oil.

FRIED RAISINS AND BANANAS

1 oz (30 g) soft margarine
1 tablespoon raisins
1 banana

Melt margarine and cook raisins gently until swollen. Add thickly sliced banana and cook a few minutes, shaking pan until hot.

MELON AND LIME JUICE

Moisten cubes of melon with a little lime juice.

BANANA SPLIT

Halve banana lengthwise and set on plate or in bowl. Pile spoonfuls of plain yogurt or cottage cheese between halves and scatter with toasted chopped or flaked nuts.

GRILLED HONEY GRAPEFRUIT

Cut grapefruit in half and drizzle with liquid honey, or top with spoonful of hard honey. Slip under the grill and cook until golden and hot.

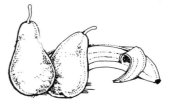

Lunches

School children have the choice of school dinners, packed lunches or coming home for lunch. Each has its advantages and disadvantages, but with nutritional foresight, you can choose what will best suit your family.

School lunch

School lunches used to be carefully planned and had by law to provide one-third of a child's caloric and protein requirements. This rule has been withdrawn and standards vary in the aims of school-meal organisers in various parts of the country. In junior schools children are not normally given a choice at meals. This is wise because less wasteful, and younger children would probably make wrong choices, opting for chips only for main course, and biscuits and sweet foods for afters. Some school meals are sadly higher in animal or hard fats and sugar than is desirable for good health, as well as lower in fibre, vegetables and fruit than is wise. This should be allowed for in planning other meals at home to ensure the total daily intake is well balanced.

Home lunch

If you have a younger child or baby it should be possible to cook a meal to suit both. Concentrate your choice of food on vegetables with meat and other protein food, and either a fruit- or milk-based pudding. All the items suggested in the packed lunch meals can also be used for your child's home lunch. Soups can be given for a hot starter (commercial soups are of very little food value so should be avoided), and this may be followed by a variety of sandwiches or other cold foods. Fresh fruit is the best dessert.

Packed lunch

Unless planned with some forethought, packed lunches can be rather high in carbohydrate and fat and somewhat low in protein, minerals, vitamins and fibre. With a little care they can be greatly superior to a cooked meal for much less than you might pay for a school dinner. Choose a good sandwich or two, or some hot food, but always accompany with some vegetables or fruit. See the charts following for other ideas.

Use your freezer when preparing packed lunches; it is an invaluable time-saver. Thaw items overnight at room temperature. Sandwiches can be frozen, depending on their filling (hard-boiled egg goes rubbery, salad vegetables lose their texture etc). Fruit jellies (not with banana), stewed fruits, and all mousses can be frozen. Vegetables and meat and vegetable soups freeze well, as do pies and flans, cut in slices and wrapped individually. Fruit loaves and cakes can be cut in slices and wrapped in freezer film, and pasties and turnovers are good lunch-box fillers from the freezer.

Lunch-box fillers
Make sandwiches from wholemeal bread which is more satisfying and contains more fibre, B vitamins and iron. White bread actually contains more calcium than brown, so while it is useful to encourage brown, it is more important to choose what will be eaten with relish. Aim in general to give a variety – rolls, French breads, etc. – to prevent boredom, or substitute with crisp breads. Spread butter and margarine very sparingly; low-fat spread, sunflower seed and low-cholesterol margarine are the best. But try using, as an alternative, peanut butter, soft cheese and soft scrambled egg as sandwich bases. Ketchup, pickle, chutney and mild mustard may be used instead, with hard cheese, pâté, or cold meats, all of which are already high in fat (although *low-fat* Cheddar is now available).

Choose a high protein food as a sandwich filling. Aim at a 60 g (2 oz) quantity of protein – one egg, two sausages etc. A scrape of meat paste or paper-thin slice of ham is not enough. Marmite, though savoury, should be used *in addition* to protein foods, not as an alternative. It is better for small children to have one well-filled sandwich as they are unlikely to have room for four slices of bread made into sandwiches.

Always make *interesting* sandwiches, or use the following ideas to fill rolls, pitta bread, plain or cheese scones.
American Ham Sandwich Spread bread with redcurrant jelly, fill with chopped ham and celery moistened with yogurt.
Pineapple and Ham Sandwich Spread with low-fat curd cheese and fill with slices of pineapple and ham.
Beef and Radish Sandwich Spread bread with cottage or soft cheese, top with sliced radish and cold sliced beef.
Sausage and Apple Spread bread with mild mustard if liked, top with layer of apple sauce and sliced sausage.

Curd Cheese, Celery and Date Use low-fat cheese, finely sliced celery and chopped dates.

Carrot, Cheese and Walnuts Low-fat curd cheese, grated carrots and chopped walnuts.

Sweetcorn, Tomato and Cottage Cheese Equal quantities of corn and cheese mixed, with layer of sliced tomato.

Scrambled Egg and Mushroom Fry sliced mushrooms in a little butter, lift out and scramble egg softly in pan.

Chicken, Peach and Cress Sliced chicken and fresh or tinned peaches with layer of cress.

Chicken Liver and Raisin Fry livers in a little oil with raisins. Chop liver and flavour with chopped rosemary. Layer with crisp lettuce when cool.

Peanut and Orange Sandwich Combine equal quantities of peanut butter and cottage cheese, flavour with grated orange rind, and moisten with a little orange juice.

Those children who are reluctant to eat meat sandwiches but like jam and have eggs for breakfast, may be tempted by the following sandwiches. To increase proteins, send with milk, milk shake, yogurt, cold sausage, fingers of chicken, cheese etc. *as well*, or some of the following recipes.

● Minced walnuts with strawberry jam.
● Curd cheese, honey and banana.
● Raspberry jam and peanut butter.
● Redcurrant jelly and minced or diced lamb.
● Cottage cheese and apricot jam.
● Peanut butter and banana.
● Date, honey and cottage cheese.
● Hazelnut chocolate spread and cottage cheese.

CRUNCHY MEATBALLS

½ lb (225 g) sausagemeat
¼ lb (115 g) minced beef
2 tablespoons fresh breadcrumbs
1 egg, beaten
1 teaspoon mixed herbs
1 tablespoon milk
3½ oz (100 g) chopped mixed nuts

Oven temperature: 190°C/375°F/Gas 5
Combine meats, breadcrumbs and half the egg. Season with herbs and beat well together. Roll into balls the size of a large marble. Dip in remainder of egg mixed with milk, and roll well in nuts. Bake for 20–30 minutes until golden. Freeze if wished.

CRUNCHY DRUMSTICKS

4 chicken drumsticks
2 tablespoons tomato ketchup
Grated lemon or orange rind
4–6 tablespoons rolled or jumbo oats

Oven temperature: 190°C/375°F/Gas 5
Spread ketchup and citrus rind over drumsticks, then roll in oats and set in oiled roasting tin. Bake 35–40 minutes. Less crunchy if frozen but may be more convenient.

LIVER LOAF

½ lb (225 g) chicken or lamb's liver
½ lb (225 g) sausagemeat
1 tablespoon mixed herbs
1 egg
3 tablespoons wholemeal breadcrumbs or oats

Oven temperature: 180°C/350°F/Gas 4
Purée or mince liver. Combine all ingredients and turn into a small loaf or cake tin. Set in roasting tin of hot water, and cover well with foil. Bake 50–60 minutes until firm to the touch in the centre. Leave to cool. Turn out and freeze, in slices if wished, or use in family salads.

KIDNEY AND BACON PÂTÉ

4 lamb kidneys
4 rashers bacon
3 tablespoons tomato purée

Halve, core and skin kidneys. Fry bacon until fat runs well. Fry kidney cut side up until golden. Turn and cook other side. Mince or purée kidney and bacon with tomato purée. Use as a spread for sandwiches or dip for salad items. Freeze if wished.

SARDINE AND LEMON PÂTÉ

1 can sardines in tomato sauce
Grated rind of ½–1 lemon

Remove tails but leave in bones and purée finely, adding lemon rind. Use as a spread or dip. Freeze for short period only.

WALNUT, DATE AND MARMALADE LOAF

½ lb (225 g) dates
¼ pint (150 ml) water
3½ oz (100 g) soft margarine
1 large tablespoon golden syrup
1 large tablespoon marmalade
3 teaspoons baking powder
4 tablespoons dried milk
11 oz (300 g) wholemeal flour
1 egg
3½ oz (100 g) chopped nuts

Oven temperature: 180°C/350°F/Gas 4
2 lb (1 kg) loaf tin

Chop dates and stew with water, margarine, syrup and marmalade. Bring to boil and simmer 2 minutes. Leave to cool. Mix baking powder and milk into flour, then add egg, dry ingredients and nuts to pan. Fold together. Turn into tin and bake 1¼ hours. Test with skewer (if damp, loaf is not ready).

FRUIT CREAM

1 lb (450 g) fruit (gooseberries, apricots, plums, damsons, blackberries, blackcurrants, etc).
2–3 tablespoons sugar
¼ pint (150 ml) water
1 sachet gelatine
1 small carton plain yogurt
4 tablespoons dried milk powder

Cook fruit, stoning plums if possible, with sugar and majority of water. Soak gelatine in remaining water. When fruit is cooked, add gelatine, stir in well and heat without boiling to ensure gelatine is dissolved. Purée fruit, when cold, and before set, stir in yogurt and milk powder. Pour into cartons and leave to set.

FRUIT MOUSSE

1 lb (450 g) fruit (strawberries, raspberries, currants, gooseberries, plums, etc).
2–3 tablespoons sugar
6 tablespoons water
1 sachet gelatine
1 small tin evaporated milk, chilled

Purée fruit with sugar if using strawberries or raspberries. Other fruit cook with sugar and 3 tablespoons water, then purée. Soak gelatine in the remaining water in small pan. Dissolve over heat and stir into fruit. Whisk evaporated milk to a thick mousse. Fold or whisk in fruit purée. Chill in pots.

Vegetables, fruit and extras

Vegetables can be either salad items to eat with the fingers, or raw or cooked, fresh or frozen, diced or grated vegetables which can be combined in a mayonnaise, yogurt or dressing, and packed in a carton to eat with a spoon. Home-sprouted seeds can add interest.

Whole fruit is best, and you can choose a wide range as they come into season. Quarter oranges and pears and apples if wished, then wrap tightly in kitchen film for transport. Home-made fruit jellies and mousses can be packed in cartons, jars or yogurt pots. Many can be made in advance and frozen.

Many children enjoy little extra items to choose from for the lunch box but these should be limited unless you are confident the more important foods are eaten. By nine to eleven years most children have fairly substantial appetites, so may need larger quantities. A 'tuck' box of goodies that your children can dip into and select what they want is a good idea, leaving you to supply the remainder if this suits all. Choose things like low-fat fruit cakes with plenty of dried fruit; biscuits low in sugar and fat, and high in fibre, containing fruit, nuts and oats; fruit loaves high in fibre and fruits; or a variety of dried fruit and nuts, wrapped in little twists of kitchen film.

Hot foods

These can be eaten with a spoon from a small unbreakable thermos (many are now available, and can be used for cold food or drinks in summer).

Hot drinks like Ovaltine, Horlicks, carob and drinking chocolate may be welcome in cold weather, or hot fruit drinks. Hot soups, if home-made, will have much greater food value, and can be made in bulk and frozen in handy-sized cartons. Thaw overnight and reheat at breakfast. Make from leftover cooked vegetables or puréed baby food with the addition of milk or stock, puréeing if necessary, and quickly reheat and pack at breakfast. Make soup for tea, family evening meal or baby's lunch, and reheat.

Hot stews – meat and chicken casseroles containing root vegetables, beans and lentils, mushrooms and red cabbage – withstand being kept hot very well. Few nutrients except Vitamin C will be lost in keeping hot or reheating. Potatoes, other vegetables and meats are best cut or diced if large for easy eating with a spoon or fork. Fish, pasta, rice and green vegetables do not lend themselves well to keeping hot. Fish toughens and exudes watery juices, pasta and rice become mushy or slimy, and green vegetables develop an unpleasant smell.

Children's choice for packed lunch

Choose one from every column. If you can eat more then choose more from any column.

| Protein | Carbohydrate | Vegetables | Fruit | Drinks |
For Growth	For Energy	For Strength	For Health	
Egg	Wholemeal bread	*Raw*	*Raw*	Milk
Cheese	Brown bread	Lettuce	Oranges	Milk shake
Cottage cheese	White bread	Spinach	Apples	(home-made)
Curd cheese	French bread	Endive	Bananas	Fruit juice (canned,
Ham	Pitta bread	Chicory	Peach	cartons or frozen
Bacon	Bread rolls	Cabbage	Pears	concentrate.
Sausage	Scones	Watercress	Apricots	Dilute to make
Peanut butter	Wholewheat cakes	Cucumber	Cherries	more thirst-
Peanuts	Rye crispbreads	Radish	Grapes	quenching if
Almonds	Plain wholemeal	Celery	Kiwi fruit	wished)
Tiger nuts	biscuits	Fennel	Melon	Tomato juice
Walnuts	Tea cakes	Mushroom	Pineapple	Squash + Vitamin C
Soya sprouts	Fruit cake	Carrot	Plums	Vegetable soup
Corned beef	Fruit loaf	Cauliflower	Strawberries	
Cold beef	Pastry	Calabrese	Raspberries	(Avoid heavily
Pork		Sprouted seeds or	Tangerines	sweetened
Lamb		pulses	Satsuma	commercial milk
Kidney pâté		Avocado		shake and yogurt
Liver pâté			*Cooked*	drinks. Add extra
Fish pâté		*Cooked*	(in jelly, mousse or	Vitamin C to weak
Sardines		(Combined in	stewed)	squash)
Pilchards		salads or soups)	Apples	
Tuna		All beans	Pears	
Salmon		Peas	Currants	
Smoked mackerel		Corn	Gooseberries	
		Potatoes	Damsons	
		Carrots	Plums	
		Swede		
		Turnip	*Fruit yogurts*	
		Parsnip		
		Beetroot	*Dried fruits*	
		Courgettes	Dates	
		Aubergines	Apricots	
		Peppers	Raisins	
		Onions	Sultanas	
		Brussel sprouts	Currants	
		Broccoli	Figs	
		Spinach	Bananas	
		Cabbage	Apples	
			Prunes	

Packed lunch menu for six weeks

Week	1	2	3
Day 1	Crunchy Drumstick Lettuce and Tomato Potato Salad Fruit Cake Squash + Vitamin C	Tomato Soup Cheese Flan Cucumber Banana	Tomato Juice Cornish Pasty Lettuce and Radish Apple

Day 2	Beef and Tomato
	   Sandwich
	Pear
	Milk
		Cheese and Pickle
		   Sandwich
		Celery
		Grapes
		Blackcurrant Juice
			Pineapple Juice
			Chicken, Corn and Apple
			   in Mayonnaise
			Watercress
			Fruit Cake

Day 3	Liver Loaf and Cucumber Sandwich Fruit Mousse Apple Juice	Crunchy Meatballs Coleslaw Fruit Loaf Orange Juice	Cream of Chicken Soup Salami in Cheese Scone Raw Carrot Orange

Day 4	Cream of Celery Soup
	Scrambled Egg and
	   Watercress Roll
	Melon
		Cornish Pasty
		Tomato
		Dates
		Raspberry Milk Shake
			Cottage Cheese and
			   Tomato in Pitta Bread
			Banana
			Grapefruit Juice

Day 5	Corned Beef and Radish
	   Sandwich
	Bean Sprouts
	Plums
	Milk
		Sardine and Lemon Pâté
		   Sandwich
		Peas and Cucumber in
		   Yogurt
		Grapes Tomato Juice
			Hard-Boiled Egg
			Russian Salad with Potato,
			   Beetroot and Cauliflower
			Grapes
			Date and Marmalade Loaf

Varied lunches are more stimulating. This plan will last for half a term, or choose favourite combinations.

4	5	6

Scotch Egg
Tomato
Muesli Biscuits
Lime Juice
	Leek and Potato Soup
	Cold Pork and Apple
	    Sauce Sandwich
	Orange
		Beef and Tomato
		    Sandwich
		Cherries
		Banana Milk Shake

Peanut Butter Sandwich
Bean Salad
Fruit Jelly
Milk
	Bacon Quiche
	Carrot and Tomato
	Fruit Yogurt
		Liver Sausage and
		    Beansprout Sandwich
		Avocado and Orange
		    Salad
		Fruit Yogurt

Cold Sausages
Celery and Cucumber
Banana or Honey
    Sandwich
Milk
	Roll with Smoked
	    Mackerel or Tuna
	Cucumber
	Peach
	Tomato Juice
		Kidney and Bacon Pâté
		Cabbage and Apple Salad
		Wholemeal Biscuits
		Milk

Cream of Celery Soup
Bacon Sandwiches
Raisins
Apple
	Cottage Cheese and
	    Minced Walnut in Tea
	    Cakes
	Dried Apricots
	Banana
	Blackcurrant Juice
		Soya Cheese and Mustard
		    and Cress Sandwich
		Carrot and Pear
		Pineapple Juice

Fish Pâté
Rye Crispbread
Tomato and Cucumber
    Salad
Apple Juice
	Cottage Cheese, Ham
	    and Pineapple Roll
	Pear
	Orange Juice
		Omelette in French Bread
		Tomato and Cress
		Satsuma
		Milk

Tea-times

Choose food that will complement those taken earlier in the day. If they have had school lunch it is wiser to presume that rather less than a good main meal has been consumed.

Many younger children, especially if they have had a school dinner, like a tea on rather traditional lines. They like tea to be tea, not dinner – a meal you eat with fingers, perhaps spoon too, but not a knife and fork job.

Whatever their desire, their *need* is for protein foods plus vegetables and fruit. If adequate meat and fish has been eaten during the day the protein may be provided by bread with yogurt, nuts, nut butters or beans and milk; pasta with cheese, macaroni cheese, cheese on toast or cheese alone; and egg dishes are also ideal unless egg was given at breakfast.

Children are unlikely to have had sufficient vegetables whether with a packed lunch or school dinner, so these should always be included. A variety of cooked vegetables with cheese sauces or grated cheese make a quick easy meal with the cheese providing protein, or a meal of meat and two vegetables can be given. Home-made soups (serve in a cup instead of a bowl, perhaps) and baked beans are both popular, and even those who like a more traditional tea can have fingers of cooked or raw vegetables which they can dunk into a protein dip.

If fruit has already been eaten this may not be an essential at tea. Most will not have had more than they need so a fresh fruit or a fruit dessert are sure to be welcome.

MACKEREL AND CHEESE PÂTÉ

1 fillet smoked mackerel
2–3 tablespoons low-fat curd or cottage cheese
Grated rind of ½ orange, or horseradish sauce

Skin and bone fish if necessary. Pound or blend to purée with cheese, then flavour with orange rind or a little horseradish. Use as spread or dip.

CREAM CHEESE AND PINEAPPLE DIP

Purée small carton of cottage cheese and pineapple, adding a little cold milk if needed.

MARMITE AND CURD CHEESE

2 oz (60 g) curd cheese
About 1 tablespoon hot milk
1 teaspoon Marmite

Beat cheese with milk and Marmite to a smooth texture.

PEANUT AND RASPBERRY DIP

2 tablespoons peanut butter
1–2 teaspoons raspberry jam
About 2–3 tablespoons hot water

Mash peanut butter and jam. Beat in enough hot water to make a smooth, soft creamy texture.

CHEESE AND CHUTNEY DIP

1 tablespoon milk
1 teaspoon chutney or pickle
2 oz (60 g) grated Cheddar cheese

Heat milk, remove from heat and add chutney or pickle and cheese. Allow to melt, and stir well, adding more milk if needed, and warm without boiling.

HOME-MADE PEANUT BUTTER

½ lb (225 g) raw plain or roasted peanuts
1 tablespoon honey
3–4 tablespoons sunflower oil

Even those children who do not like the tacky expensive commercial nut butter are likely to love this real peanut spread. Grind nuts in coffee mill, blender, food processor or mincer. When finely ground add honey and oil. Bind to a rough but relatively smooth texture (which will depend on the machine you use). Store in fridge to maintain good flavour.

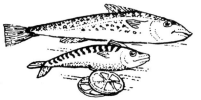

VEGETABLES FOR DUNKING

Raw	*Cooked, Hot or Cold*
Carrot	Carrot
Courgettes	Parsnip
Celery	New potatoes
Crisp lettuce	Corn on the cob
Fennel	Cauliflower
Strips of raw cabbage	Beans
Tomatoes	Broccoli
Cucumber	Calabrese
Radish	
Sprouted seeds or beans	
Avocado	
Endive	
Chicory	
Watercress	
Mushrooms	
Cauliflower	

YOGURT

1 carton UHT milk
2 tablespoons dried milk
1 tablespoon fresh yogurt

No special equipment is necessary. Warm milk until just tepid. Stir in dried milk and yogurt – this may be reserved from last batch you made (but buy new starter yogurt regularly for best results). Store in a very warm place in original carton unless thermos or yogurt-maker used.
- 2½–3½ hours in wide necked thermos.
- 4–5 hours at back of Aga or on radiator or in large bowl of moderately hot water.
- 5–7 hours in container in slow cooker with water around. Cover with cloth *not lid*.
- 6–12 hours in a cylinder cupboard.
- 6–12 hours in yogurt maker.

The quicker a set is achieved and the yogurt immediately chilled the better the flavour. Times are approximate but using a yogurt-maker gives the sourest yogurt and a thermos the sweetest. Make sure your mixture does not over-heat or the yogurt will make curds and whey (use for making scones, bread or cheese – freezing until convenient to use).

Tea-time entertaining

By five years – often indeed by three – children have developed quite a busy social life and enjoy going out to tea with friends or having them in. Sadly many otherwise intelligent mothers allow their own children and encourage the children of their friends to develop very bad eating habits. Only squash, or worse, pop, is provided to drink. The tea table contains buns, chocolate and other biscuits and crisps etc., and cake followed by commercial jelly, ice cream and probably sweets. Any sandwiches are likely to be ignored with these temptations, and no fruit or vegetables are offered. It is an appalling way to feed children, but many are eating like that regularly during the week or even demanding a tea of this type daily.

DO very severely limit the quantity of crisps etc., if these are given.

DO allow *only* one cake, bun or biscuit for each child so that other foods are eaten from hunger, or alternatively, do not put on the table until children have had time to eat other food first. For children under and around seven, make these items in sweet cases, tiny cake cases etc.

DO offer milk and fruit juices or combine fruit juice with fizzy drinks. If you have a Sodastream real fruit juices can be carbonated or mixed with soda water.

DO provide vegetables – sticks of carrot, cucumber, celery, pieces of lettuce, cress, quartered tomatoes and radishes.

DO provide fruit. Colourful dishes of oranges cut into wedges, satsumas, apricots, whole and quartered apples, pears and peaches (dip in fruit juice to prevent discoloration), pineapple chunks on sticks, bowls of separated grapes, raspberries, strawberries to eat with fingers.

DO provide protein foods – quartered hard-boiled eggs, cubes of cheese, ham, spam and sausages are popular on sticks. Provide nuts with caution – peanuts at an exciting occasion are a risk.

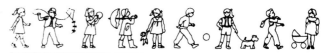

Preparing their own meals

For the seven- to eleven-year-olds, this is an important part of learning about food – and life. Even the most reluctant meat eater will consume with gusto the chop he has grilled himself! Make sure the meals he or she prepares are based on the three-point plan below. You can supervise unobtrusively, and let them help prepare casseroles and cook vegetables when time permits at weekends and holidays. Kneading bread and rolling pastry is fun but more valuable is the knowledge of how to put food together to make a meal.

Children of seven to eleven should not be left cooking unattended in the kitchen since many activities could be potentially hazardous. An atmosphere conducive to good concentration by all is most important for both child and parent. Do not have radio, television or the rest of the family providing distractions. While it will always be quicker to cook the food yourself 'unhelped', unless children have experience they will never learn to be of use and to feed themselves.

Make them understand that *at every meal they should eat:*

● A high protein food (meat, fish, cheese, eggs, milk or soya).
● Fruit and/or vegetables, preferably both, and fresh.
● Cereal food, preferably whole-grain (good whole-grain breakfast cereal, wholemeal bread, brown pasta, brown rice, whole-wheat crackers, or beans).

Encourage them to choose good breakfast cereals and serve these with plenty of milk or plain yogurt. Serve a washed fresh fruit or fresh or grilled tomato, or fruit juice. A simple cooked breakfast of eggs, fish, cheese or meat etc.

Encourage them to prepare packed or simple lunches (see packed lunch ideas earlier in the chapter). Many ingredients will need preparation only, not cooking. Remember to serve foods from each group.

Encourage them to choose grilled foods for speed or foods that only need heating (beans). Even learning to wipe the tin, opening the tin, then emptying contents and pushing lid into empty can for safety, is important training.

Eat what your body needs

The following paragraph and the page opposite should be read – and appreciated by – the children themselves.

Just as a car needs petrol, oil and water to work properly so our bodies need fuel and water so they may move and work. Our bodies also need to grow and be repaired, so fuel and water alone are not enough. Our bodies are made of what we eat and drink. We must remember this every time we put something in our mouths. We should not eat only for pleasure, we should eat what our bodies need, too. Many foods and drinks look nice and taste good but are bad for our teeth or health and do not provide what our bodies need. These foods we should avoid.

Fuel

All food provides fuel for our bodies to give us warmth and energy. We measure the amount of energy in a food in calories. Those calories we do not use we store as fat. Fats and oils in our food contain the most calories. Sugar and starchy foods like cakes and biscuits are also high in calories. We must not eat too much of these because we will become fat. Other foods will provide the fuel we need and *also* help us grow, keeping us strong and healthy.

Protein for growth

It is needed like the bricks in a house to build the growing body and to repair it. Protein is very important for growing children, and should be eaten at every meal, particularly at breakfast.

High Protein Foods	Lower Protein Foods
Milk	Beans, especially baked beans
Eggs	Nuts, especially peanuts
Meat	Breakfast cereals, especially
Fish	wheat and oat cereals
Cheese	Bread and pasta

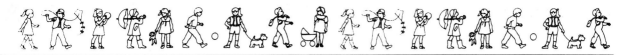

Calcium and phosphorus with Vitamin D for strength

These minerals are needed for strong bones and teeth, and they need Vitamin D to help them.

Calcium	Phosphorus	Vitamin D
Cheese	Nuts	Sunshine on our skin
Milk	Wheat and oats	Cheese
Yogurt	Liver	Milk
	Milk, eggs	Butter or margarine

Vitamin A for good health

Needed for a healthy skin and eyes and to protect the wet surfaces of the eyes, nose and lungs.

Liver	Carrots	Melon
Eggs	Spinach	Apricots
Herrings	Parsley	Plums
Mackerel	Watercress	Tomatoes
Tinned fish	Sweet potato	Peaches
Butter	Broccoli	Prunes
Margarine	Pumpkin	Tomato juice
Milk	Lettuce	Orange juice

Iron with Vitamin C for health and strength

Iron is needed for the blood which carries oxygen round our bodies. It is also helped by Vitamin C. Without enough of both we feel tired, and cuts and bruises do not heal quickly. Vitamin C is also very important as it helps protect us from infections and keeps us healthy. Cooking food destroys some of the Vitamin C so eat some raw fruits and vegetables every day.

Iron	Vitamin C	
Liver	Broccoli	Blackcurrants
Meat	Brussel sprouts	Oranges
Eggs	Cabbage	Gooseberries
Wheat and oat cereals	Cauliflower	Strawberries
	Tomatoes	Melon
Wholemeal bread	There is a little Vitamin C in
Dried fruit	potatoes, other vegetables and
Dark green veg.	all other fruit

B vitamins for good health, growth and strength

These are needed for good appetite and to make you lively and happy.

Thiamin	Riboflavin	Nicotinic Acid
Wheatgerm	Liver	Peanuts
Liver	Cheese	Liver
Kidney	Mushrooms	Chicken
Whole-grain cereals	Eggs	Bacon
	Milk	Mushrooms
Pork	Yogurt	Wholemeal pasta and bread
Ham and bacon	Beans	
Nuts	Lentils	
Bread	Meat	Peas
Flour	Peanuts	Baked beans
Brown rice		Jacket potatoes

Fibre and fluid for health

Waste products in our body must be got rid of quickly to keep us clean inside and feeling fit. This is helped by eating foods that are not heavily refined, and which contain the natural skins and fibres of grains – wholemeal bread, etc – fruit and vegetables.

We need to have plenty to drink as well. Choose 1 pint (575 ml) of milk each day and some real fruit or vegetable juice (not squash); also drink about two glasses of plain water.

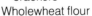

Wholemeal bread	Dried fruits	Baked beans
Whole-grain cereals	Apricots	Corn
	Prunes	Peas
Wholewheat pasta	Berries	Lentils
Brown rice	Currants	Jacket potatoes
Wholewheat crackers	Unpeeled fresh fruits	Green vegetables
Wholewheat flour		

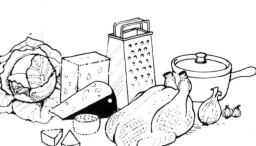

Chapter Seven
Feeding sick children

Information in this chapter is to supplement any medical treatment and advice, and explain further the meaning of giving 'plenty of fluids' or 'a light diet' (see end of chapter).

The earliest possible return to the enjoyment of food is what every mother will want for her children after the normal childhood illnesses. Modern treatment will mean most of these are, fortunately, short lived and a few days without food will do little harm. Nevertheless a high daily intake of liquid, more than 3 pints (1.5 litres) is recommended for most of the childhood infections, and giving a well balanced diet each day is of considerably less importance than ensuring enough fluid is taken. Appetite is rarely lost for long enough to cause concern, but a little information as to what to offer for different illnesses may save time and trouble.

Antibiotic treatment

Most often given to small children for ear and some throat infections. Some antibiotics may cause slight upset of the stomach, even diarrhoea, as the natural bacteria of the gut which aid digestion can be affected. Yogurt taken regularly throughout the period of treatment may help some children. The appetite is usually affected by the illness as well as the treatment, so offer small quantities of favourite foods that are low in fat and easy to digest; fruit jellies, poultry, white fish or egg dishes, tiny sandwiches, home-made soups, ripe or cooked fruits. Give plenty to drink: a wide variety of juices, squashes and milk drinks should ensure a good total intake.

Common cold

Small children may expect to get three to seven colds a year, especially when they or an older brother or sister starts school and the germ is regularly picked up and spread round the family. A normal intake of Vitamin C daily (45 mg) will not prevent this. Very high doses – 500–1000 mg of Vitamin C as ascorbic acid in powder form – are believed by some to be helpful in preventing colds if taken at the earliest symptoms.

Extra care in scalding all cups and utensils used by the cold sufferer may help in preventing the spread round the family and, more important still, used paper handkerchiefs should be promptly burnt or flushed away and the hands washed, particularly before touching food.

A small baby with a cold will have great difficulty feeding if his nose is congested. He cannot breathe and suck simultaneously and will become very frustrated, lacking both nourishment and the comfort of sucking whilst he is unwell. When your baby has a cold check before he wakes for a feed to see if he is showing signs of having difficulty in breathing through his nose. A few drops of oil of eucalyptus, Karvol or a dab of Vick placed on a tissue (not on the baby's face) then tucked under the bottom cot sheet below the baby's nose, will give off vapours which will help clear the congestion in about 15 minutes. Small frequent feeds may be the best policy if breast-feeding to comfort the baby and to ensure plenty of fluid. For a bottle-fed baby offer extra fruit juice or boiled water in addition to what milk feed he is happy to take.

Fruit may be the only welcome food for a child with a heavy cold; an older child will be able to clearly express his preferences, even if it is for jelly at breakfast. Purées of fruit and tinned or cartons of juice may be set with gelatine and purées of vegetables quickly turned into soups with chicken stock and a little fruit juice. Cooked puréed tomato or carrot with stock and orange juice makes a quick and excellent soup. As the weakened sense of taste will make many foods seem dull, remember to season well and strengthen the flavour by adding herbs, lemon, orange or pineapple to meat and fish dishes to make them more tempting. Serve very small portions. Eating with a cold can be slow and uncomfortable, and a large plateful a daunting prospect. Several very small courses may be much more attractive. Start the meal with a little fruit juice, then a small bowl of soup followed by a little fish or chicken in a good sauce, plus vegetables, then fruit jelly or a juicy fruit.

Constipation

It should be diet, not drugs, that will cure this complaint in infants, children and adults, unless a doctor recommends otherwise. The amount of dietary fibre and fluid taken may need to be permanently altered to assure the comfortable passing of stools. Each individual's requirements will be different, but basically it is a slow passage of waste through the body, and a lack of fluid and fibre which reduces water content of the stools and makes them hard.

In babies it is of no consequence whether stools are passed three times a day or once every three days, as their bowel habits fluctuate. It is only important that these should be *comfortably* passed. For most babies the giving of boiled water first thing in the day will be the best remedy, especially for bottle-fed babies. Home-made purées of any fruit or vegetables will also help, as they contain more dietary fibre than commercial refined products. Give them without added cereals or sugar (or salt, under eight months).

In fully breast-fed babies constipation is unlikely, and if it does occur it may be caused by *under-feeding*. This can also be the problem with bottle-fed babies, as some infants need larger feeds than recommended for the average child. Babies can vary as much in their requirements as adults, so try offering larger feeds to see if this helps.

For toddlers, children (and adults), choose the right foods to start the day. Whole-grain cereals are high in fibre and include muesli, porridge and the whole-wheat cereals such as Weetabix, Wheat Flakes, Shredded Wheat, Shreddies, etc. Bran cereals are very high in fibre – the best being natural bran – but other bran cereals can be used on their own or with other cereals. Corn and rice cereals are not a good choice, especially the sweetened varieties, which are highly refined and have insufficient fibre. A fried breakfast and fruit juice alone is a poor choice as well, unless a whole-grain cereal or bread is also eaten.

'Brown' bread is a vague term: whole-wheat, wholemeal or high bran varieties should be chosen as much as possible. The same is true of biscuits: rye, oat or whole-wheat are a better choice. If in addition to this plenty of fresh fruit (better than fruit juice for breakfast) and vegetables are served, there should be no need to spurn a few more refined foods occasionally.

Beans, prunes, figs and other dried fruits make excellent natural cures for constipation. For babies, give just the juice of prunes or figs, as dried fruits may prove too strong a purge for those under two years old. Increase the intake of water, not milk (unless under-feeding in a small baby is suspected), cut out eggs for a few days, and keep the intake of fat low. Add ½ to 1 tablespoon of natural bran to the diet each day, 1 teaspoon for babies over seven months. This can be stirred into purées, yogurt, meat dishes or cereals, whichever is the most palatable.

Cot death

This all-too-frequent tragedy is included because many have claimed it was due to modern bottle-feeding. As it has been recorded since Biblical times, there is obviously no specific present-day cause. Bereaved parents may be questioned on the feeding of their baby, but this is meant in no way to imply criticism or fault, but rather to help in the statistical research: this shows that infants have been fed a very wide range of foods even from the earliest days of their lives, and although this is not now recommended for a variety of reasons, cot death is *not* one of those reasons.

The tragedy strikes a large number of infants between two weeks and two years, but the most common age is four months, which coincides roughly with an introduction to solid food. A mother would be mistaken in imagining she had given inappropriate foods.

Breast-fed babies are at less risk of respiratory infections which in some cases have been thought to be a contributory factor. Breast-feeding, nevertheless, cannot be considered a protection.

Incorrect mixing of bottle feeds with too much powder may cause dehydration and a baby to become ill, but this will *not* cause the sudden death of an apparently healthy baby (the characteristic of 50 per cent of cot deaths). Symptoms of illness should always be checked with a doctor, especially if your child is around four months.

Bereaved parents may wish for support and reassurance from the Foundation for the Study of Infant Deaths (see Appendix).

Fever

If your child has a temperature it is unwise to encourage him to eat, so give a little food only if it is asked for or as he recovers. Plenty to drink to replace lost body fluid is essential. Choose non-milk drinks such as water, fruit juices and drinks, clear soup, chicken stock or Bovril. The more he can drink the better, so tempt your patient with a wide variety of these at regular intervals. If he is feeling chilled, a warm drink will be more welcome; if hot and flushed offer cold but not chilled drinks (a large quantity of chilled drinks in a feverish child can cause tummy ache). Remember not to take the temperature orally after cold or hot drinks or you will get an inaccurate reading.

Fainting

This is not caused by anaemia, but can be caused in some children by bad eating habits. Those who miss out on breakfast or go too long without food may be prone to fainting. This is most likely to occur if children have to stand in stuffy crowded places like buses or school assembly. Ensure your child has breakfast every day and that he is aware that on school outings etc. he must eat at regular intervals.

Do not give a child food or drink if he/she is about to faint, is unconscious or has just regained consciousness. Wait a minute or two, and when the child is fit to sit up and hold a cup, offer a sweet drink.

Gastroenteritis and stomach upsets

This may be caused by allergy, food poisoning, or by a virus. Children may develop diarrhoea as a result of bacteria from tonsil, ear and urinary infections. In older children diarrhoea can also be caused by anxiety.

For most forms of diarrhoea the treatment is to encourage the patient to take plenty of fluid and give solid food only if asked for. Small children may not understand the difference between tummy ache and hunger, so generally it is wise to avoid food.

The loss of fluid is potentially very dangerous in infants. Contact your doctor promptly if your baby has both diarrhoea and sickness, if diarrhoea is severe, or if baby is not taking plenty of boiled water or frequent short breast-feeds. Your doctor may wish to see the baby quickly or advise special feeds which only he can prescribe. With mild diarrhoea reduce

the strength of the bottle feed or give water, but seek professional advice if only water is given for more than twenty-four hours. Omit solid foods for baby until milk feeds are again taken normally and there is no sign of diarrhoea.

As the patient recovers the best foods to offer first are boiled rice, cooked carrot and banana. Follow this with yogurt or toast, then other easily digested foods low in fat and not too acid. A clear soup of chicken stock with rice and diced carrot boiled in it is quick and easy, or try diced or mashed banana and yogurt. A refreshing Indian drink is yogurt with water; this will be easier to digest than cow's milk, so may be offered to toddlers and children who are recovering from stomach upsets. White fish, chicken, milk, eggs, bread and cereal are good to follow. Keep all servings small: they are more tempting and the stomach needs time to recover slowly. This may take several days.

In small babies damage may be done to the intestines during gastroenteritis which may not then function efficiently. Return to normal feeding carefully and slowly. Contact your doctor if you are concerned or if your baby's stools do not return to what was normal for him, or if there is a return to diarrhoea. Occasionally a baby may develop an allergy to a particular food he was able to eat before his illness.

Halitosis or bad breath

This is not caused by constipation as was often formerly thought, so changing to a high-fibre diet will not help. The most frequent cause in children is dental decay. Some children will also have halitosis with tonsillitis even when the tonsils are only slightly infected.

Any signs of a strange smell on a new baby's breath should be reported to the doctor immediately. It may indicate an enzyme deficiency in the digestion, the most common cause being phenylketonuria which all infants are checked for in the first few days. Infants with these deficiency diseases require a specially formulated feed which will prevent a build-up of poisons.

Where halitosis has no obvious cause it may indicate a diet deficiency of Vitamin B_6, especially if accompanied by tension, wind, indigestion, headaches and dandruff or other such mild indispositions.

Brewer's yeast tablets, wheatgerm, beans, bananas, peanuts, sweetcorn and citrus fruits in the diet may improve these conditions as well as improve the general health.

Mumps

The salivary glands are inflamed in mumps, and this may cause great discomfort in eating, drinking and even thinking about food! Acid foods and drinks – orange, pineapple, lemon, grapefruit, blackcurrant, gooseberry, tomato, vinegar and ketchup – are especially likely to cause some pain. Stiffness of the jaw may make chewing uncomfortable, so diminishing the choice of food still further.

If the child has a temperature you will be giving aspirin every four hours. Dissolve in a very little water, milk, rosehip drink, barley water, apple juice or Lucozade, or give the medication in syrup form. Within half an hour this will also act as a painkiller, and is the ideal time to offer drinks which are less acidic. Warm chicken stock or broth or drinks of Bovril will cause least discomfort.

A baby with mumps should continue to be offered breast or bottled milk at feeds. He will need extra fluids – boiled water, rosehip or apple juice – if his temperature is raised. If sucking is causing discomfort, you doctor can advise on a painkiller to give half an hour before a feed; liquids may be offered on a spoon or in a cup if sucking remains difficult.

As soon as the child is interested in food, plenty of skimmed milk drinks and soft foods that require little chewing are a good choice. Meat, fish and vegetable soups will be nourishing and easy to take (although tomato may cause discomfort). Bread to dunk in soup will soften and be easier than toast.

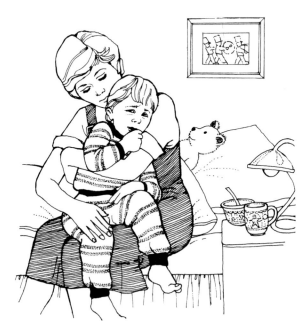

Scrambled eggs, mashed potato, milk puddings, custard and jelly will all slip down easily while chewing is still painful.

For breakfasts avoid crunchy cereals; try porridge or Weetabix soaked in milk. For fruits try raw banana, kiwi or avocado, peeled and mashed. Try also pears and stewed eating apples such as Cox or Sturmer which are not as sharp as cooking apples. Fresh ripe apples, pears and melon may be given grated to a pulp. Give vegetables boiled, steamed and puréed (only tomato is likely to cause any discomfort), and finely chop or mash poultry and white fish (both low in fat) until the patient can enjoy normal meals again.

Other glands may also be affected by mumps, though not often in children. It is nevertheless wise to keep the intake of fats low. Use skimmed milk and avoid butter or margarine when you start to give food, to give the body time to recover.

Intake of sugar and sweets should also be kept to a minimum. Sucking of sweets will in any case be uncomfortable so discourage well-meaning friends and relatives. With inflamed salivary glands, the teeth will quickly become coated with plaque and very vulnerable to decay. Regular and frequent brushing of the teeth and rinsing of the mouth with water to keep the mouth clean is advisable.

Sore throat

Chilled drinks can often numb the pain, which is especially helpful before eating. If food is unwelcome, ice lollies are bound to be popular. Freeze fruit juices; yogurt with fruit purée; banana mashed with milk; honey mixed with egg yolk and milk. Dip in hundreds and thousands as you serve. Freeze segments of orange on a toothpick; serve home-made ice cream too. Give soothing warm drinks of honey, lemon and a little glycerine if you have it. Spoonfuls of honey to suck at two- to four-hourly intervals will aid the healing of the throat. Choose smooth, easy-to-swallow food like soups, macaroni cheese, minced chicken or fish with creamed or mashed vegetables, or scrambled egg.

Travel sickness

This usually occurs in cars, coaches and boats, but can even result from playing on swings and roundabouts.

Infants who are drowsy, cold, clammy and pale when travelling are the most likely to develop travel sickness. In the young you may have no advance warning so it's wise to be well prepared, and check their colour regularly. Give little to eat before and during travelling, preferably drier foods, and keep drinks to a minimum just before and for the first hour of a journey. Some travelling mums find wine gums, peppermint or ginger biscuits quite helpful for mild travel sickness. For most children it is important to look out of the window, not down at a toy, book or game, which increases the rolling sensation. Tape recorders (with ear phone in public transport) may be a useful distraction. A doctor or chemist can advise on suitable travel pills according to age.

Hot soup or a hot drink will help a child recover more quickly from the chilled feeling which may remain at the end of a journey.

Vomiting

Most babies will regurgitate or posset a small amount of food and this is of little consequence. More serious vomiting in a new-born baby must be promptly checked by a doctor. Some babies continue to vomit quite a large part of each feed although there is nothing clinically wrong with them, so your doctor may recommend thickening the baby's feed. Ensure that your baby is not allowed to cry for too long before a feed as a lot of air may be swallowed, and keep the baby upright in a baby chair or sling for a while after feeds or place a pillow or cushion *under* his mattress at the head of the pram or crib so that he is less prone. If he continues to gain weight, there is usually little cause for concern.

Vomiting in babies, toddlers and children may mark the beginning of an infection, even a simple cold: it may be caused by migraine, travel sickness, food poisoning, gastroenteritis or whooping cough. Vomiting does not normally last more than six to eight hours. If a baby is sick as long as this it is wise to consult your doctor. In an older child seek professional advice if after twelve hours no fluids are being kept down.

Maintaining and replacing lost body fluids is important, especially in the very young. Breast-fed babies should be fed little but often, and if they have difficulty in keeping down any fluid and also have diarrhoea, ring the doctor; meantime try water.

Bottle-fed babies who are having difficulty keeping down small milk feeds should be offered a little water very frequently; again contact your doctor if the condition is serious and continues for more than a few hours. Once a baby is able to keep down water, give a very diluted milk feed, one-quarter feed and three-quarters boiled water. Proceed to half feed, half water, and gradually return to normal. Do not give any solid foods or unmodified cow's milk until your baby is drinking normally.

Be ready for baby's posseting with tissues, towel or apron to protect your clothes. Do not put plastic bibs on baby in his cot or pram because of the danger of suffocation, but place absorbent towel or napkin under the baby's head – this can then be removed without unduly disturbing him. Regurgitated food is not unpleasant smelling, but may be mildly sour.

When true sickness occurs, dust clothes, carpets etc., with bicarbonate of soda to remove odour, then clean with disinfectant in cold water. Soda-water solution or dry bicarbonate may be used for the removal of any smell. If sickness is caused by food poisoning or infections, prevent contamination spreading by a very high standard of hygiene.

For toddlers and older children the quick return to normal fluid intake is also important. Small sips of fluid are easier to keep down than larger quantities, and drinks are best at room temperature, not chilled. Although neither can normally be recommended as a healthy drink, both Pepsi and Coca-Cola may be much easier to keep down than water if your child (or you) is vomiting. The drinks should be flat, not fizzy, so pour from a height and stir briskly. They are cheaper and much more readily available than Lucozade which could also be used, and particularly useful if you are travelling abroad and uncertain of local water.

Salts and potassium are lost in sickness and diarrhoea. As soon as the patient is able to take fluids, these can be replaced by giving warm drinks of chicken broth or stock, Bovril or Marmite, and fruit drinks (choose the least acidic first).

When the child again wants food choose those that require little chewing at first. Chewing may cause the child to start retching again.

Whooping cough

This can be a long illness, and if whooping and coughing cause the child to be sick, a few precautions can be taken to ensure this is minimised and as much food kept down as possible to prevent the child or baby becoming very weak.

To minimise coughing fits, breast-fed babies may be put to the breast at the onset of a bout of coughing; this may help prevent vomiting as well as exhausting coughing. With bottle-fed babies, older infants, and children the best time to give drinks and food is immediately after a spasm of coughing. This will give the maximum amount of time for food to be digested before the next bout of coughing, which may cause sickness.

Food and drink for the sick child

Taking plenty of fluids implies that a child needs at least 2–3 pints (1–1.5 litres) of fluid a day or as much as he may be comfortably encouraged to take. Even for a common cold extra fluid is needed by the body and when a child has a fever more body fluid is lost through the skin than normal to reduce the body heat by evaporation. Many children with a fever may feel too ill to demand the extra fluid they need so it is part of good home nursing care to ensure a child is encouraged regularly (every half hour or hour, whenever awake), to take a few sips of a suitable drink.

No child who is ill should be pressed to eat, only tempted. There are two important guidelines. The first is that food should be given in very small quantities to begin with; only gradually increase this quantity, as many childrens' eyes are bigger than their 'stomachs at this stage, and they can very easily and quickly reject food after the first few mouthfuls. Others' natural instincts are not so reliable as usual, and they may eat *too much* if offered a lot of tempting food, and then regret it half an hour later. The second important point is that the food offered in such sparse quantities should be food that is easy to digest. This does not mean foods should be sweet or starchy (likely to be cloying and to contribute little to a child's recovery), nor should they be fatty, fried, red meats, or very fibrous vegetables. Sausages, pastries, burgers etc. should also be avoided. Offer eggs, white fish (poached or steamed) and chicken with potato, carrot, cauliflower, fruits and bread when milk puddings and light soups and other drinks are not enough.

Chapter Eight
Special diets and special needs

From preference or necessity, you may need to choose a special diet for your children if you are confronted with problems.

Overweight

Your heart was designed to pump blood round your body at its ideal weight; whether large or small framed, your heart was designed specifically for that size of frame. But if you carry around a greater weight than you should – if you are *over* your ideal or natural weight – your heart will be under unnecessary strain, and this will shorten its working life.

If a baby is 3–4 lb (1.3–1.8 kg) overweight at one year it is as if he were moving around with six to eight packets of butter. He will be considerably hampered in his movements, there will be slower hardening of his back bones, and his soft leg and feet bones are likely to bend from carrying weight for which they are not designed. This can cause permanent damage to the back, legs, feet and joints, creating a variety of problems throughout life.

Overweight babies and children tire quickly, becoming short of breath. They are predisposed to asthma, bronchitis, and other chest ailments. In later life they are more prone to emotional disorders and diabetes. The heavy folds of flesh will chafe, causing skin infections, and could result in eczema.

Babies are not born overweight, but even by six weeks some infants are heading towards obesity as babies, children and adults. We are born with a number of fat cells, go on to make additional fat cells in the first year of life particularly, and can continue to make them throughout our lives. When excess weight is gained the fat cells inflate as fat is deposited and more fat cells made.

Children most at risk of being overweight are those with overweight parents. If *both* parents are overweight, the child has a four to one chance of being fat. If one parent is overweight, the child has a fifty-fifty chance. In both these cases overweight is caused by the normal eating patterns of the family concerned being inappropriate for their needs. Inherited life style can be *much* more influential than genes. Another example lies in children who are handicapped or subnormal. They are often inactive, and have very low calorie needs, but are frequently given unsuitable food as an expression of love or consolation for their misfortune. And bottle-fed babies may be given bottles made up with just a little extra powdered formula. This causes too fast a weight gain plus a thirst which is often mistaken for hunger and more food given. Not all fat babies become fat children, but quite a lot do. Controlling obesity in children is *very* difficult so early prevention is vital.

Our inherited shape, metabolic rate and potential for retaining deposits of brown fat after infancy all affect how many calories each of us need.
There are three basic physical shapes:
Ectomorph Long limbed with narrow hands, fingers and feet. Least likely to become overweight.
Mesomorph Well proportioned body, has to balance energy expenditure with calorie intake to maintain good weight.
Endomorph Short limbed, broad feet and hands with stubby fingers. Has to take the greatest care to control weight throughout life.

The metabolic rate – the natural rate at which the individual uses energy – depends on the above physical shapes to some extent. Exercise and temperament will also play a part as we can *raise* our metabolic rate by choosing to be more lively and energetic. The brown fat theory is relatively new. We are said to be born with deposits of this special fat and that the more we have and retain through childhood the more efficiently we burn excess calories. We turn them into heat which the body can rid itself of instead of converting the excess calories into fat deposits. It does not appear to be possible to deliberately alter our brown fat.

The overweight family

In a family at risk of members becoming overweight it is important that a much more positive view is taken of the need for fewer calories. No one complains that a mini car is much cheaper to run because it needs less fuel than many other cars, and this should be the attitude to feeding a family who have low fuel requirements! Instead of feeling deprived, they should be grateful that they don't have to spend a fortune on food!

Choose food for the family with low calorie requirements carefully. Aim at those that are rich nutritionally, which contain high quantities of vitamins and minerals, as only small quantities will need to be served. Choose those foods low in fat but high in fibre (brown bread and jacket potatoes do not have to be omitted). Avoid buns or generous spreadings of butter or margarine. Avoid chips and roast potatoes. Serve white fish (without batter or coating) as well as chicken, liver, kidneys and other lean meats. Limit sausages, burgers and bacon. Serve beans, including baked beans, peas and lentils which are high in protein, fibre, vitamins and minerals. Base puddings on a wide variety of fruits with a minimum of sugar or fat.

Take a positive line when you want to indulge your low-calorie family. Treat them to super fruit: a peach, tangerine, punnet of strawberries or raspberries, a fresh pineapple, a kiwi fruit or extra pear or banana. Or to a special vegetable such as asparagus, globe artichoke (great fun for children but do not dip in butter), fresh peas and good tomatoes. Choose special meat – a nice lean chop or kebabs – not fatty mince, pies, burgers and sausages. These will all bring pleasure to those who like food too well!

The overweight baby

Breast-fed babies may put on weight very quickly in the first three months, but if solely breast-fed you don't need to worry about this. Weight normally levels off later in the first year, and these babies can be safely fed on demand until four months. Bottle-fed babies who are putting on weight at more than a normal level may well be becoming overweight unless they had a particularly long frame at birth. Weight gain is never at a steady rate but needs to be compared over several weeks and months. At your baby clinic your child's weight will be plotted on a chart, and you will be told of too big a weight gain.

A trap many mothers fall into, is that of jiggling baby up and down towards the end of a feed to rouse him to finish the last of his bottle. When he's no longer really interested, leave those last drops and throw them away. Over-filling at each feed is a very bad habit for life. And do remember that bottle-fed babies are likely to need a little water daily (about 2 fl. oz or 50 ml).

At around four to five months infants may cry more, and you should not automatically presume this is hunger. A baby of this age needs entertainment and activity, so if he cries two to three hours after a feed do not allow to breast-feed or bottle-feed *again*, but plan another activity – play with him, use a baby bouncer, push in a pram, take shopping or visiting friends. By this age food should not be the only interest and pleasure offered.

When weaning between four and six months, only *very small* tastes of food should be given. Avoid most commercial baby foods. Choose a good commercial baby cereal and give once a day only, then make all fruit and vegetable purées *without sugar* for other meals, offering cheese, eggs, meats and fish at recommended ages.

As the child is weaned, from the ages of seven to twelve months, guard against overweight with the following:

The overweight baby

DO make food progressively lumpier so that quantities are not gulped down. Give plenty of finger foods, not too many purées

DON'T give any sugar, sweetened cereal, cakes, biscuits and sweet rusks.

DON'T give commercial fruit yogurt. Add unsweetened fruit purée to plain yogurt.

DO keep fats to a minimum, and use cottage in preference to hard or cream cheese. Choose poultry and white fish, not fatty mince. Avoid oil, butter, lard, margarine etc., in cooking.

DO restrict milk intake gradually to 1 pint (575 ml) daily as food intake increases. Three meals a day plus 1½ pints (850 ml) milk is too much for infants by eight to nine months. Choose other drinks with care – unsweetened fruit juices are best.

The overweight toddler and child

DO avoid sausages, chips and pastry.

DON'T give sugar, biscuits, cakes or sweets. Give ice cream rarely, make fruit and yogurt ice lollies instead.

DO give fresh fruits and vegetables and use these for a between-meal snack if necessary.

DO give higher bran cereals – Weetabix, Readybrek or, better still, those that need some chewing such as Grape-Nuts or Shreddies.

DO plan better low-calorie meals for all the family, with *no* chocolate sauces, sponge puddings or pastry.

DO restrict milk to ¾ pint (425 ml). If skimmed milk is needed because of severe overweight remember to give Vitamin D supplement.

DO use smaller plates so smaller helpings look generous.

DO make sure there is plenty of chewing time at each meal.

DON'T use convenience foods (except baked beans), as most are high in calories, low in fibre, nutritionally unsatisfactory and too quickly eaten.

DO use foods of high nutritional value so small quantities will satisfy all nutritional needs.

DO remember three chocolate digestive biscuits contain 400 calories. *This is more calories than a meal consisting of 7 oz (200 g) jacket potato/4 oz (115 g) white fish with lemon juice/4 oz (115 g) tomatoes, green vegetables or cauliflower/either an apple, 4 oz (115 g) strawberries or a banana!*

DO watch what drinks your child chooses. Squash and pop disguise many calories. Your child should drink *water* at least twice a day. Very weak tea or coffee can be given unsweetened.

DO use artificial sweeteners for children set in bad habits, but it is better for health to avoid sugar and chemical sweeteners altogether.

General guidelines for overweight

Never presume that he or she will grow out of puppy fat. Act immediately there are signs of chubbiness. Hold the weight steady by altering the child's diet and limit his overall intake.

It is an act of gross unkindness to allow your child to become fat and the butt of ridicule from other children. Boys are particularly unkind to Billy Bunters and girls may be spiteful to fatties too. Fat ten- to eleven-year-olds are often tall for their age but do not feel reassured that they will become slim as they grow quickly in their teens. On average they stop growing much earlier, growing little after twelve for girls and thirteen to fourteen for boys.

Always weigh a child regularly at bathtime (every home should have scales) and keep a written record with the date. Check each fortnight or month. Check height as well and compare on growth chart (see Appendix 1). Ideally, only those children who are on the upper level for height should be on the upper level for weight; children of average height should have average weight. Some girls tend to become chubby at around eight to twelve but most lose this weight by seventeen plus. Those who become anorexic in their teens, however, are likely to have been chubby when younger, so it is vital to monitor weight and diet at around eight to twelve to prevent the risk of later obsessive – and very dangerous – dieting.

Seek medical help and advice promptly if you feel you are not controlling the situation. Your aim is to keep the weight steady while the child grows, *not* for the child to actually lose weight unless a doctor recommends this because of severe obesity. Encourage plenty of constant activity, running round the house on errands or active lively play inside or out, not sitting in front of the television.

Control pocket-money spending. Make all children in the family keep a notebook of how they spend their pocket money if you suspect it is being spent on sweets etc. Low-calorie chewing gum only may be a good compromise, or put a large percentage of pocket money in an account at the Post Office for enforced weekly saving so that larger amounts can be withdrawn for a specific purchase – and keep daily temptation at bay.

Inform *all* relatives or friends who might give unsuitable edible gifts and insist on their complete cooperation. Allow an Easter egg at Easter but otherwise avoid all chocolates and sweets etc. Ask them to give a tangerine or other fruits only.

Include plenty of food in the diet that needs a lot of *chewing*, such as raw vegetables, fruits and nuts, whole grains and meat that has not been ground into burgers, mince or sausages. Chewing is good for everyone, and it ensures that the food is not gulped down quickly, when *more* would be eaten. Some people also need *oral* satisfaction in their meals; they like the sensation of food in their mouth just as they may have enjoyed thumb sucking etc.

Always remember that it is a *kindness* to deprive your overweight child of unsuitable foods or the large quantity of food he craves – and cruel to allow him to become fat. Show your love and concern by giving more of your time, and help him to develop interests that will take his mind off food and lead to a healthy active life.

Underweight

Some babies and children are perfectly healthy on well below normal weight. They may have inherited a light frame or maybe are shorter than average. Some are always very skinny with ribs clearly visible, and may look particularly thin as toddlers. They may or may not have good appetites. Ensure plenty of good food is available but do not pressurise children to eat. Skinny children are often very healthy.

Tiny or erratic appetites

Ensure children take recommended vitamin supplements and in addition plenty of B vitamins to stimulate appetite, either as supplements, or Vitamin B rich food – liver, kidney, other meat, milk, eggs, beans and well chosen breakfast cereal. Do not *urge* child to eat as this may be counterproductive and off-putting. Ensure *only nutritious foods and drinks* are available. Let him have as much and any of these as he is keen to eat.

It is very common for a small child to eat only one good meal every few days or so, and to pick at food with little interest at other times. Do not work on the principle that you would rather your child ate anything rather than nothing. He is *more* likely to be

malnourished if he eats sweets and biscuits which need protein, vitamins and minerals to digest them than if he has nothing. All children will eat eventually from pure hunger, even if this is erratically. Make sure there is a good choice of his most favourite *nutritious* foods about, and *absolutely no* opportunity to eat even one mouthful of junk food, squash or pop. See Faddy Toddlers, Chapter Five. Avoid any coercion, pressure or bribery. If it appears to be a matter of indifference on your part whether your child eats or not at a meal, he is unlikely to create meal-time tantrums or be deliberately uncooperative.

Ill-health

After a series of colds and minor illnesses, especially in winter, many children seem to have a poor appetite and are very thin. Concentrate on foods rich in B vitamins rather than sweet or rich fatty foods which will dampen poor appetites. Offer plenty of small meals of well chosen foods. Do not offer crisps, biscuits and sweets: their need is for proteins, vitamins and minerals, so tempt with fruits, homemade fruit ices and other nutritious foods.

Malnourished children

Malnourished children may show one or more of the following symptoms: a difficult temperament; dark rings round somewhat hollow eyes; a pronounced pallor; a tendency to infections of the throat, chest, skin and stomach; and poor quality of hair and fingernails.

Malnourishment can be caused by a problem in the digestive system, and this is usually noted in the first year. Infants who have any odour in their breath (unless they have been eating garlic!), intermittent or perpetually loose stools (except in the first months of breast-feeding), or those whose stools are pale and very offensive, smelly, foamy, fatty or in any way irregular, should be checked by a doctor. Long-term disorders of the digestive system can upset the absorption of nutrients so that additional vitamins and minerals may be needed. Advice from doctors and hospital dieticians on foods must be followed exactly since food which is unsuitable for him can prevent proper absorption of nutrients from suitable foods.

The diet of infants and children with food allergies needs careful balancing. Inform your doctor or clinic if you are planning to take a child off milk or wheat or a large range of foods long term, as this can lead to an imbalance in nutrition and you should have expert advice on supplements if these are needed. Omitting eggs, fish or citrus fruits can be adequately compensated for on a normal diet.

Malnourishment can be caused simply by bad eating patterns. This is very common when weaning and until children reach five to seven years. Adequate quantities of food are consumed so far as calories are concerned, but this food could be totally inadequate in quality. Quality does not refer to expensive ingredients as most of the cheapest ingredients, if correctly prepared, are very rich nutritionally. Cut out all junk food. Offal and chicken are some of the cheapest meats. Baked beans, dried beans and soya are even cheaper. Fresh and dried milk, plain yogurt and eggs are excellent value, and are labour-saving protein foods rich in vitamins and minerals, with no additives. Bread is a useful source of protein, cheaper and much better for health than biscuits and cake. Jacket potatoes, pasta and brown rice are cheap and highly nutritious. Carrots and cabbage are invariably cheap. Give fresh fruit and vegetables in season.

Vegetarian and other diets

Vegetarian publications are unlikely to give you a totally unbiased view, but leading nutritionists in Britain and the USA consider that while too much animal fat and animal protein is undoubtedly consumed for good health in general, a completely vegetarian diet is *not ideal* for an expectant mother.

It is probable that the diet given to vegetarian infants is not always adequate for seven to twelve months while they are being weaned and have very high nutritional needs. Fussy and faddy toddlers are also difficult to feed an adequate diet during the period of one to four years. Make sure there is plenty of milk, cheese and eggs in the diet in the early years. Choose the most highly nutritious breakfast cereals, those fortified with riboflavin (B$_2$) and nicotinic acid, but not too high in bran. Give ground peanuts for extra nicotinic acid. Use plenty of soya flour and other soya products which, along with eggs, will ensure adequate iron. Make sure proper vitamin supplements are taken daily of A, D and C and that highly refined and junk foods are kept out of the diet.

If you are a determined vegetarian it is important that you do not concentrate on what you will *not* eat. You must plan very carefully instead what you *will* eat, so that you can compensate adequately for a diet

without meat, fish or poultry. Even if not a committed vegetarian, a good vegetarian dish at least once a day is an excellent choice for good health, and a much wider use of pulses, fresh vegetables and whole-grain foods can only be beneficial.

It is important that expectant mothers and children under three to four years consume the correct proportions of all the essential amino acids which are the constituents of protein foods. Protein is supplied by foods in the following listing for a vegetarian diet and, as can be seen, soya is by far the richest source, higher in fact than meat or fish.

Expectant mothers require 2 oz (60 g) protein per day and small children about 1 oz (30 g). A high proportion of complete proteins is particularly valuable at these times to ensure optimum growth and proper development of the foetus or child so that the brain size reaches its potential, and the general health of the child will be good.

The protein intake can be made up to the optimum total with incomplete proteins from textured vegetable protein (TVP), as well as all beans (other than soya), peas, lentils, nuts, grains and cereal products (bread, pasta and flour). These are required in greater quantity to provide useful protein. Only about half the protein value can be well used so they are best not considered the major protein foods of the day during pregnancy and early childhood.

In addition to a diet high in complete protein the vegetarian's diet needs to be high in wheatgerm and in fresh green and yellow vegetables – carrots, peas and corn – which are normally a good source of zinc. This mineral is not well absorbed in vegetarian diets and it is known to contribute to infertility, congenital malformation, premature birth, poor growth, anaemia and poor lactation. Zinc can be absorbed

Vegetarian Protein Sources	
Source	Protein, g per 1 oz (30 g)
Eggs	3.4
Cheddar cheese	7.2
Cottage cheese	4.3
Milk	.9
Yoghurt	1.4
Skimmed dried milk	10.2
Wheatgerm	7.4
Soya 'grits', low-fat	13.5
Soya flour	11.0
Dry soya beans	10
Soya beans, fresh and reconstituted	3.0

through the skin so infants will take in some from zinc and castor oil cream on their bottoms! Vegetarians would be advised to take supplements of zinc before and during pregnancy and to give zinc to their children in childhood, especially during the early years.

Vitamin B_{12} is provided in only small quantities, by eggs, milk and cheese. Insufficient causes a specific anaemia. The early symptoms are masked by the ample supply of folic acid in the vegetarian diet. A supplement of Vitamin B_{12} is advisable for all vegetarians during pregnancy to ensure that adequate iron is absorbed and deposited in the baby for his first months of life.

Vegetarians usually need to spend more time in the preparation of good imaginative food than meat eaters, and need to give greater care to creating a well balanced diet for their family. Highly processed commercial vegetarian foods will not be as rich nutritionally as foods in their raw or natural state and, as with every other kind of processed food, labels should be read for they may contain unnecessary additives.

Soya flour and soya beans are somewhat unpalatable hence the growth of the novel protein industry. Choose foods of soya in preference to field beans which are not as rich nutritionally. Proteins may also be extruded as TVP, used mainly as meat extenders in normal diets and 'spun' to simulate different cuts of meat popular with vegetarians. TVP is a good substitute for meat except that it is lower in zinc, Vitamins B_1, B_2, and B_{12}, available iron, the essential amino acid found in meat protein, called methianine, needed for growth. Eggs as well as peanuts, milk, and cheese will all help to create a well balanced diet.

Children and meat

Many children, both young children and teenagers, can become very sensitive to the idea of eating animals. This distaste is very natural in the many children who are imaginative or sensitive to the feelings of others – admirable qualities in themselves. It requires the greatest tact and care in the presentation of meat in their diet so as not to offend them. One vegetarian in the family is a nuisance since it is not sufficient for them to eat family meals and leave out the meat.

Really good substitutes are essential for growing children. If you notice a child becoming sensitive about meat, plan some good vegetarian dishes each week for all the family. When meat dishes are being served, choose those in which the meat is partly or

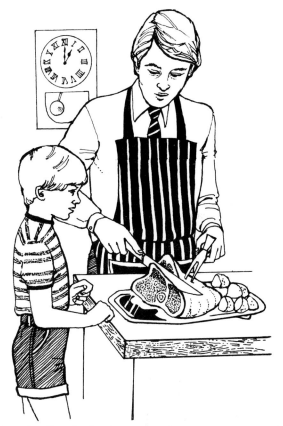

largely disguised – lasagne, mince, sausages, meatballs, pâté and stews where animal forms or bloody meat juices are not evident. Whole chickens, legs of lamb and pink meat juices conjure up alarming images in the minds of young children, so always be aware of this. If they *are* served, do not place them on the table in front of a sensitive small child, but carve or put on a plate out of sight. An invented *name* for the dish can sometimes help.

There are many small children who do not like meat because they are very lazy about chewing. If food is made too easy for them to swallow from seven months onwards they never learn the art of chewing. Food should not only become progressively firmer in the first year but should continue to require more and more chewing for the next two to three years so that children do not expect to just swallow items down effortlessly. Give foods that require most chewing at the beginning of a meal when they are really hungry and prepared to work to satisfy hunger. The continental custom of giving meat and sauces first, followed by a vegetable dish then dessert, is a good ploy here: try giving the meat first, then when a reasonable amount of meat has been eaten (about 2 oz or 60 g), serve the softer vegetables.

Indigestion

If just changing to a vegetarian diet, the sudden introduction of pulses can cause a lot of indigestion. Begin gradually and build up the quantity slowly. Some people find beans easier to digest if not served with high carbohydrate foods such as bread, flour, potatoes or rice. Many herbs aid digestion, especially savory – called the 'bean herb' – which is similar in flavour to sage. Winter savory is very easy to grow in the garden. Sage, mint, parsley, dill and fennel all aid digestion, and are good with beans.

Allergies

The vegetarian diet may not suit some people with allergies. If your baby or child has eczema, asthma or other allergies and you suspect that his condition would be better without milk, cheese or eggs (common causes of allergy), it would be wise to consider very carefully whether the vegetarian diet you have chosen for yourself is in fact ideal for your child. Seek as much help as you can from allergy societies or qualified dieticians in working out a new and appropriate diet.

Vegetarian cookery

Vegetarian food can look rather dull in colour and largely brown. Ensure attractive, tempting food in some of the following ways.
● Garnishes of tomatoes, watercress, lemon, orange and other fruits.
● Use plenty of herbs and mild spices, and sprinkle dishes with chopped parsley.
● Use colourful ingredients – fresh or tinned tomato, red kidney beans, green flageolets, carrots, red, green and yellow peppers, black aubergine.
● Top dishes with grated cheese, sieved egg yolk, spoonfuls of yogurt or soured cream, olives, chopped nuts or vegetables.
● Serve some raw fruit or vegetable at every meal for more texture.

The recipes which follow look good, taste good *and* do good!

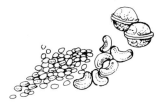

PEANUT AND SOYA MEATBALLS

| 1 onion |
| 2 tablespoons oil |
| 6 oz (175 g) unroasted peanuts |
| 1 egg |
| 2 tablespoons soya flour |
| 5–6 tablespoons wholemeal breadcrumbs |
| 1 teaspoon mixed herbs |
| Salt and pepper |

Oven temperature: 200°C/400°F/Gas 6

Finely chop onion and fry in oil until golden, then cool. Grind the nuts, then stir into onion with egg, soya flour and sufficient breadcrumbs to make a firm mixture that will roll into balls. Add herbs and seasoning. Shape mixture into balls the size of whole walnuts. Bake in the oven on a greased baking tin for 20 minutes. Serve with a tomato, mushroom or cheese sauce. The mixture may also be made into burgers.

MUSHROOM AND NUT CASSEROLE

This recipe is suitable for any infant over eight months who can eat mushrooms.

| *Base* |
| 7 oz (200 g) ground nuts |
| 3½ oz (100 g) wholemeal breadcrumbs |
| 3 tablespoons soya flour |
| ½ teaspoon dried thyme |
| 2 tablespoons sunflower margarine |

| *Topping* |
| 12 oz (350 g) mushrooms |
| 2 tablespoons sunflower margarine |
| 1 tablespoon flour |
| ½ pint (300 ml) milk |
| ½ teaspoon salt |
| Pinch nutmeg |
| ½ lb (225 g) cottage cheese |

Oven temperature: 190°C/375°F/Gas 5

Combine nuts, breadcrumbs, flour and thyme, and turn into ovenproof dish. Dot with margarine and bake for 10–15 minutes. Meanwhile wipe the mushrooms, slice thickly, and fry very quickly in fat until golden. Stir in flour, then milk and seasoning. Bring to the boil. Spoon first cottage cheese then mushroom sauce over nut base and bake for further 20–30 minutes. Garnish with watercress.

EGG AND ONION GRATIN

2 medium onions
2 oz, (60 g) margarine
6 eggs, hard-boiled
1 rounded tablespoon flour
1/2 pint (300 ml) milk
Salt and pepper
3 tablespoons grated cheese

Oven temperature: 200°C/400°F/Gas 6

Peel and slice onions, and cook gently in half the fat in a covered pan. Peel eggs, halve, and separate yolks and whites. Slice whites, place in bottom of 1¾ pint (1 litre) ovenproof dish. Tip over the onions and add remaining margarine to pan. Allow to melt then stir in flour. Remove from heat, add all the milk, and stir well until smooth. Bring to the boil and season to taste. Press yolks through sieve with your thumb, one at a time, and scatter over onions. Spoon over sauce to cover contents of dish. Sprinkle on cheese and bake 20 minutes. Serve with hot crusty wholemeal rolls and a tomato or green salad.

Suitable for babies over seven months.

BEAN AND CHEESE PILAFF

1 medium onion
2 tablespoons oil
7 oz (200 g) brown rice
1 medium tin tomatoes
1 pint (575 ml) vegetable stock
1/2 teaspoon salt
1 teaspoon savory or marjoram
4 oz (115 g) broad beans
4 oz (115 g) green beans, sliced
4 oz (115 g) beansprouts
4 oz (115 g) cottage cheese
3 oz (90 g) Cheddar cheese, grated or diced

Chop onion and fry in oil until golden. Stir in rice, tomatoes, stock, salt and herbs. Cover and cook gently until liquid is almost absorbed and rice tender (about 35–45 minutes). Add broad and green beans, and when lightly cooked stir in beansprouts. Allow to heat through then lastly stir in the cheeses.

Suitable for babies from seven months.

HAZELNUT AND LEEK FLAN

Filling

1 lb (450 g) leeks
1½ oz (40 g) margarine
1 rounded tablespoon flour
1/2 pint (300 ml) milk
1/2 teaspoon salt
1 large egg

Pastry

4 oz (115 g) wholemeal flour
1½ oz (40 g) margarine
1 oz (30 g) white vegetable fat
2 oz (60 g) ground hazelnuts
1–2 tablespoons water

Oven temperature: 190°C/375°F/Gas 5
7 inch (18 cm) flan tin

Wash and trim leeks, slice thinly and cook slowly in fat in covered pan for 7–10 minutes. Remove from heat, stir in flour then milk. Bring to boil, stirring well, and simmer for 5–6 minutes. Season then leave to cool.

Make pastry by rubbing fats into flour until like breadcrumbs. Stir in nuts and enough water to make a firm but not crumbly dough. Roll out and line flan tin. Beat egg into cold leek sauce, turn into pastry case, and bake 35–40 minutes until set in middle and pastry golden. Serve with salad and jacket baked potatoes.

Suitable for babies after eight to nine months; filling only from seven months.

Vegans

The Vegan diet – which is not only vegetarian but will allow *nothing* of animal origin, so no milk, cheese, yogurt, eggs, etc. – is inadequate during pregnancy and early childhood without additional synthetic supplements. Adequate protein can easily be supplied by sufficient soya and wheatgerm, which can be backed up with nuts, beans, peas, lentils and whole-grain foods, but the diet is likely to be a poor source of calcium, iron, iodine, riboflavin, B_{12} and Vitamin D.

Your doctor should be advised if you wish to remain on a Vegan diet while pregnant. It is important that you should be referred to a hospital dietician so that you can together plan a diet with any essential supplements given to ensure your own health and, much more important, that of your future child. He will be at greater risk of a number of mineral and vitamin deficiencies which can cause problems.

In Vegan families babies should be breast-fed for at least the whole of the first year of life. Nut and soya milks require synthetic supplements to assure sufficient calcium, other minerals, vitamins and the correct balance of essential fatty acids and amino acids. While in theory a Vegan diet can meet most of a child's nutritional needs, in practice it is quite difficult to achieve a diet sufficient in calcium, Vitamin D, riboflavin, Vitamin B_{12} and also calories for energy. Children on Vegan diets have normally a lower weight (not necessarily a bad thing) and also a lower height than average. If the child's bones have not reached their optimum size because of too low a level of Vitamin D and calcium, the skull and brain may not have reached their potential either. It is most important, particularly for infants under three or four years, that the greatest care is taken in planning an adequate diet.

Macrobiotic diets

Any diet that is largely based on a very narrow variety of foods will not be wholly adequate, particularly during the critical period of growth of the foetus and young child. Ensuring the correct provision of essential vitamins, minerals and other nutrients is rarely possible on a limited diet without the addition of appropriate supplements. A hospital dietician can give the best informed advice for those who choose limited diets after discussing with you your normal intake of food or that of your child. Keep a detailed daily report for a week before going so that a proper appraisal can be made.

Those who follow these diets without expert nutritional advice and the modification of their diets with correct supplements during pregnancy and a child's early life are at great risk of having a miscarriage, a premature birth, a complicated delivery, a baby who is malformed, or a child who does not reach his full mental and physical potential. Adults on limited diets planning to become parents should ask for expert advice *before* they conceive. It is important that both future father and mother should not have nutritional deficiencies at the time of conception. Miso, a Japanese soya bean product, is often much favoured in diets of this nature, but it is *not* suitable for expectant mothers, infants or small children, because of its high salt content. The fermentation process it undergoes makes it unsuitable for infants.

Bircher Benner diet

This is a partially, though not wholly, vegetarian diet where only small quantities of fish, meat, and eggs are eaten. This is combined with the excellent rule that half the daily food intake should be of raw ingredients (all meals should begin with them): salads, raw fruit (fresh or dried), nuts and raw grains (those that are only crushed or rolled). These last ingredients are used in the famous Bircher-Muesli which contains a wide variety of grains, nuts etc. that have not been exposed to heat or processed in any way that would damage nutritional value. Dr Bircher Benner died in 1939 and was the forerunner of the present interest in healthier diets with greater stress on the benefit of foods not deprived of their natural nutritional value. He advocated cutting out of the diet tea, coffee and alcohol, and his diet still provides excellent guidance for expectant mothers and children today.

High fibre diet

In principle this is a very healthy new diet, which is ideal for adults and all but the youngest children. It is unwise to take this high fibre diet to severe extremes as there is considerable reduction in the absorption of some minerals and vitamins where much fibre is present. For small children raw bran and very high-bran cereals are too great a purgative and prevent proper absorption of nutrients. This could damage their healthy development, so only a moderate level is desirable for them. During pregnancy a mother may feel confident that she is eating all the right things, but a high bran intake could disguise malnutrition as a result of poor absorption. If you plan a very high fibre diet to lose weight, return to a moderately high fibre diet for a few months before you plan a pregnancy.

Special needs
Diabetes

Only one in twenty sufferers of diabetes develop the condition in childhood. Diabetics are unable to produce sufficient insulin for their needs and, in the case of child diabetics, must receive precise quantities of insulin by injection, which must be carefully balanced with their food intake and energy output. Children and their parents will be trained in the proper management of the condition by a local specialist and dietician, and their advice must be very carefully followed throughout childhood to ensure the diabetic can live a normal, active, and healthy life.

Diabetes is often inherited, especially the possibility of late-onset diabetes. The child diabetic becomes thinner and drowsy, is thirstier than in the past, and more frequently passes urine. If these four symptoms are combined, it is wise for your child to see the doctor. The number of children with diabetes now doubles in the UK every ten years.

There is an increased risk of a child developing diabetes if either or both parents were consuming a very high level of nitrates in their food around the time of conception. Excessive use of fertilisers in modern farming can cause a high level of nitrates in vegetables, particularly sprouts and cabbage, and nitrates may also be leeched into the local water supply. But the major source is in processed and cured foods, particularly ham and bacon. If diabetes runs in the family, it would be wise for potential parents to choose a low nitrate diet to reduce as far as possible the risk of a child inheriting the disease, or causing damage to the foetus which could later result in diabetes.

It has been known for many years that while a few diabetics develop the disease in childhood or as teenagers, most of the remainder develop the disease because they are overweight. They may produce a normal amount of insulin, but it is insufficient for their overweight body and bad eating habits. Tablets of insulin can be used for these sufferers but slimming to a normal body size and maintaining a suitable sensible diet will make these unnecessary.

The new findings linking diabetes with nitrates and greater care in maintaining an appropriate weight with good eating habits could considerably reduce the number of diabetics in the future. Those who risk inheriting a tendency to diabetes should be particularly careful to avoid overweight.

The greater interest in fibre in the diet has resulted in the realisation that plenty of fibre slows the absorption of sugar and starches in food so that there are not such sudden heavy demands made on the body's production of insulin. Diets for diabetic children and adults now stress this need for fibre which allows a somewhat greater freedom in the choice of food. For more information, contact the British Diabetic Association (see Appendix II).

Autism

Autistic children are particularly difficult to feed, but they need a specially nutritious diet, with all the B vitamins, especially B_6 and A, D, C and E. Adequate protein and linoleic fatty acid (sunflower seed and corn oil, chicken and pork fat) are important to minimise their problems.

Since good cooperation is unlikely it is wise to have no highly refined and junk foods readily available. Natural hunger can then only be satisfied with foods of good nutritional quality: meat, fish, eggs, nuts, cheese, milk, bread, fruit and vegetables. Vitamin and mineral supplements are a good idea if the diet appears in any way inadequate.

Mentally handicapped

These children should not be relied upon to demand only what they really need in their diet. They may need much encouragement to eat a carefully balanced diet, and particular care should be taken that they do not add overweight to their other problems.

Pyloric stenosis

A fairly common problem especially in boys between four to twelve weeks where the muscle at the outlet of the stomach tightens and narrows the stomach exit. Feed is forcibly thrown up in violent vomiting leaving the baby hungry. The baby remains apparently fit and healthy at first but he gradually becomes dehydrated and weak from hunger if the condition is not eased.

The treatment normally offered is medicine to relax the stomach muscle 15 minutes before a normal feed and if this does not stabilise the condition, a simple and very effective operation is performed.

In America some babies have been treated by supplementing their normal feeds with ½ to 1 tablespoon of uncooked wheatgerm mixed with a little milk feed every hour during the day for three to four days to see if the extra B vitamins and minerals will cure or ease the problem. It would be wise to consult your doctor before attempting this as you need to have your baby's condition confirmed and, of course, monitored very carefully if he is unwell.

Chapter Nine
Allergies

Allergies are adverse reactions to items that are eaten, drunk, inhaled or touched. The substances causing food allergy are often proteins.

In small babies, especially under four months and up to about seven months, the immature digestive system does not function efficiently, and food may not be broken down properly before being absorbed. The body's reaction to foreign proteins in the blood-stream may be to produce antibodies. In about one child in five very large amounts of a special antibody are produced. These may become fixed to cells in the mucous lining of the nose, sinuses, lungs, digestive system, or to the skin. When the infant is next exposed to a substance to which it has produced antibodies, allergic reactions will occur, causing a possible lifetime of problems.

Atopic is the name given to the large number of people whose bodies over-react to produce large amounts of antibodies and, as a result, develop symptoms. Parents who are atopic have a 50 per cent chance of passing this sensitivity on to their child, although the child may not have the same symptoms, or to the same degree. The most common are eczema, asthma and hay-fever; less common are migraine, or stomach upset, causing sickness, stomach cramps, diarrhoea, or bloated stomach. Other reactions include urticaria, allergic dermatitis, conjunctivitis, catarrh and croup.

While individuals may have only one allergic complaint, they may suffer from several. Some allergies may be outgrown, while others do not commonly afflict the young. Those who are atopic may also show severe reaction to insect bites or an allergic reaction to certain drugs. The reaction may be to the drug itself, or because it has been cultured in its production with eggs (a common allergen). So discuss family allergies with the doctor before your infant's immunisation programme begins.

Much interest is now being shown in establishing whether hyperactivity is also an allergic condition, and whether other forms of mental disorder can be linked to the diet.

In all allergic conditions, food, drink, or items touched or inhaled will be only one factor contributing to the onset of an attack. The emotional state – whether the sufferer is tired, distressed, anxious, over-excited – also plays a part in determining the severity of a reaction: at times of family crisis, excitement before a happy occasion, when not fit because of colds or other minor infections, or when taking exams, the reaction may be much more severe. At other times, the condition seems to largely clear up and the sufferer seems less sensitive to a food or other factor which had previously triggered an attack. As symptoms wax and wane for no specific reason, satisfactorily isolating foods which trigger allergic reaction can prove difficult and often needs the help of an allergy specialist and a dietician.

Foods which cause allergy

While almost any food or drink is capable of causing an adverse reaction in specific individuals, there are fortunately a few main culprits. This makes the guessing game of what food is upsetting a baby or child from amongst the hundreds of ingredients he consumes straightforward in most cases, irrespective of the symptoms. Top of the list come *cow's milk*, *cheese* and *eggs*. Other foods frequently causing allergy are *fish*, *wheat*, *citrus fruits* and *chocolate*. More recently, it has become evident that many are allergic to the wide and ever-increasing use of artificial food colouring and additives. Many of these foods form the basis of normal meals and leaving them out of the diet may lead to an unbalanced diet, so the following may prove useful.

Looking for alternatives

Allergen	Alternative Foods
Cow's milk	Goat's milk may be preferable, or soya and nut milks. Allergy will also include cheese, yogurt, butter and cream and other dairy products, ice cream, and commercial foods containing whey. Soya products resembling cheese are available at health-food shops. Some brands of margarine do not contain whey (all list contents). Oils and white fats can be used in baking and cooking. Ice creams may be replaced by water ices. Milk is a valuable source of calcium and Vitamin D, which is needed in large quantities in pregnancy, lactation and childhood. If no substitute is consumed a calcium supplement should be discussed with the doctor and Vitamin D always taken in winter (all year for dark skins).
Chocolate	Not essential in the diet, but a popular flavouring. Use carob, which is available in health-food shops, for drinks, desserts and baking.
Fish	Use meat and pulses as replacement protein. Shellfish are particularly likely to cause allergic reaction.
Artificial Food Colouring and Additives	Natural food colours or their synthetic equivalents are less likely to cause a reaction and are used in butter, cheese, and brown bread. Choose beetroot, turmeric and paprika to colour food at home. Synthetic dyes and additives are used in most commercial food products such as soft drinks, packet soups, jams, cakes, puddings, ice creams, biscuits, tinned peas, sausages and burgers. Some additives are known to cause allergic reaction. The following are not recommended for infants or young children, and are high risk for those with allergies: E102, E104, E107, E110, E120, E122, E123, E124, E127, E128, E132, E133, E150, E151, E154, E155, E210–220, E250, E251, E310, E311, E312, E320, E321, E621, E622, E623, E627, E631 and E635.

Allergen	Alternative Foods
Eggs	Serve liver or kidney regularly for a balanced diet. Many cakes, teabreads, gingerbreads, buns and biscuits can be made without eggs. Use a thin paste of flour and water brushed on before crumb-coating fish, meats and fritters. In some cases only the egg white causes allergy or small quantities used in baking are insufficient to cause a reaction. Give egg white *well* cooked not soft, as in cooked custards, and soft scrambled egg. Cooking well may inactivate the substance causing allergy, and will be better tolerated. Avoid soft meringue, ice creams and mousses with uncooked egg white.
Wheat	As in flour, bread and many cereals, it is usually the gluten content which causes allergic reaction and this is present in wheat, rye, oats and barley. Rice is the best alternative grain to use as a first cereal; maize and millet are also gluten-free. Rice Krispies, or cornflakes can be used for breakfast. Sago, tapioca, cornflour, arrowroot and potato flour are of little nutritional value, but useful in cooking. Brown rice is the best alternative to wheat in the diet, being also a source of bran and B vitamins. Some individuals allergic to wheat are able to tolerate rye, barley or oats, but this should only be tried under medical supervision for coeliac sufferers (coeliac disease is a special type of gluten allergy).
Citrus Fruits	Rosehip syrup, tomato and blackcurrant juices, as well as apple and pineapple, are excellent juice alternatives, the first three being very rich in Vitamin C. Choose from a wide range of other fruits for desserts or in cooking.

Reduce risk of allergy in your baby

A greater understanding of the cause of allergies has resulted in a change of ideas on what foods are suitable for babies, especially in the first four to seven months of their lives. In some of the research, it appears that careful avoidance of certain foods in the first months of mixed feeding may reduce the risk of a baby developing allergies by 30 per cent, and the baby may hope to have better health throughout childhood.

Parents who have themselves suffered allergies and whose children are, as a result, at greater risk of developing them, should take the greatest care to follow up-to-date advice on feeding their babies. With as many as one in five children expected to develop an allergy, views on infant feeding have been revised radically in the last few years. The greatest care during the first months of life may seem tedious, but it is more than worthwhile, since seven months of care is miniscule compared to the years which can be spent sorting out special diets for older children, teenagers and adults.

Human milk is able to create a protective lining which coats the infant's gut to give some protection from the proteins that are not broken down properly in an infant's immature digestive system. This is invaluable in the first two weeks and remains of great importance for the first four to six months of life. As a result, specialists advise all mothers, *especially* those who have themselves suffered allergies, to breast-feed as long as possible, preferably with no topping up, or addition of cow's milk formula. It is hoped that this may greatly reduce the incidence of allergic reaction.

To further reduce the risk of allergy, foods should be very carefully selected in the first seven months of life, and introduction to solid foods delayed until at least four months, preferably five to six months if possible, and thereafter introduced slowly with great care.

Cow's Milk Breast-fed babies should if possible be given breast milk alone for seven months. Try to avoid all cow's milk, cheese, yogurt, etc., until then. Where baby is bottle-fed, discuss with your doctor the possibility of using soya or goat's milk as an alternative to the modified cow's milk normally used.

Citrus Fruits Choose rosehip, blackcurrant and tomato juices, or just the ascorbic acid (Vitamin C) available in powder form, particularly if there is a history of allergies in the family.

Cereals Rice is now strongly recommended as the only cereal from four to seven months.

Eggs Egg white carries a greater risk of causing reaction so you are advised to give yolk first.

White Fish This is usually given from seven months. Serve only a small quantity the first time. Shellfish are not recommended for a variety of reasons until two years.

Pulses Peas, beans and lentils may cause allergy in some, so give root and leafy vegetables before introducing these.

Nuts Not recommended before seven months, even finely ground.

Chocolate Chocolate is not recommended in the diet of infants and small children.

Artificial Food Colours These are not added to commercial baby food and should be avoided as much as possible in home-prepared food (custard powder, for instance). As a wide range of foods suitable for general consumption – fruit, yogurts, jam, biscuits, ice cream – are introduced, parents should be aware of the large range of artificial dyes and other additives which are present and which might cause some adverse reaction.

Feeding the atopic family

If attempting to establish a correct diet for an allergy sufferer leads to a tense atmosphere at meals, much of the advantage of a more suitable diet may be negated. The tension alone can trigger an allergic attack. Creating meals that will suit all is preferable to pointing out all the goodies on the table which are 'forbidden fruits' to one member of the family. It often happens that more than one member of the family has food allergies, and with luck they may overlap in their intolerances to, say, eggs or milk and cheese. Where they do not share the same reactions to foods, it may be essential to offer alternatives at meals eaten by all.

While special food can be prepared and served to suit just the allergic baby and toddler, by two years old most children will need to be fed with the family with the minimum of fuss and extra work for their mothers. At breakfast, a range of cereals and juices can be offered to suit the preferences and needs of each member of the family. When considering cooked breakfast, it may again be wise to be flexible; give eggs, or fish to those that can take it with grilled or fried tomatoes and bacon, kidney, beans, rissoles, sausages to those who are allergic to fish or eggs. For small children, a daily cooked breakfast is not always necessary.

When it comes to main meals, it is always best to strive to serve dishes suitable for all. For main dishes, avoid cheese, beef or pork if any of these cause a problem. Lamb, chicken, rabbit or turkey rarely cause allergies, so include the offal of these for full nutritional benefit – liver, kidney, tongue, heart and sweetbreads. If gluten is not tolerated, always thicken sauces and gravies with cornflour, arrowroot or potato flour. Few vegetables cause allergy and if a variety is always served, everyone can be accommodated without any member of the family being deprived.

If you are giving a pudding, serve a selection of fresh fruit to all regularly to save trouble and time. To make a pudding only some members are allowed to enjoy is bound to cause friction. Fruit jellies made from fruit juices or thin fruit purées, set with gelatine (1 sachet to ¾ pint or 450 ml fruit juice or purée) make desserts ideal for most with allergies. Pies and crumbles will also be suitable. Suet puddings or shortcakes can be made instead of sponge puddings containing eggs if these have to be omitted. Goat's milk yogurt may be tolerated by those allergic to cow's milk products, and is a great asset in making desserts where it can often replace cream.

When an allergy sufferer is a guest at a friend's house, it is wise to inform his hostess, especially if it is for a lunch or dinner or overnight stay, to save any problems of embarrassment. Do not just give a list of things he can't eat – no milk, eggs or fish – which can be offputting for the hostess. Say instead what *is* suitable: 'any fruit or vegetables, except peas and beans' or 'he will bring his own milk for his breakfast cereal'.

When allergic children are attending parties, it is wise to let them decide whether to say 'I'm sorry I can't eat egg sandwich, I'm allergic', or 'no thank you, I'm allergic' (which they can manage even at four years old, and will receive sympathetic help from a hostess), or to taste and enjoy the chocolate cake and blow the consequences. Even that four-year-old can make this decision and understand he may suffer. He should not be greeted at home with an 'I told you so' reaction, but instead, a cheerful but sympathetic 'I'm sure it was delicious' from Mum who makes a mental note to give a suitable medication later. He should then be able to enjoy visiting friends without being over-anxious which alone can cause a flare-up of something like eczema.

It is quite possible for children and adults to suddenly become allergic to a food which was previously enjoyed when commercial prepared foods are being consumed. A new additive or different type of food colouring may be the cause, but it is quite possible to eat eggs, for example, for many years and *then* develop a sensitivity. Alternatively, a food may not be tolerated for several years and then can be enjoyed without any adverse reaction. It is therefore wise not to expect to have to give up a food for life, but check tiny quantities at intervals, when the skin and general health are good.

Eczema

An allergic skin condition where the skin becomes red, swollen and itchy with small blisters developing on the surface. These weep when scratched and become crusted before healing, to leave the skin thickened, scaly and very dry. (The blisters should not be confused with milia, the tiny pearly or yellow spots that occur on a baby's face in the first weeks of life. The skin in this case is not reddened and spots are caused by blocked sebaceous glands in the immature skin. They disappear naturally in a few days or weeks.)

In a baby, the cause is usually a reaction to some food eaten, and the cheeks or eyelids, or round the mouth, develop a rash, or rashes occur at creases at the wrist, elbow, behind knee, at neck or in the nappy area. Contact with wool or synthetic fabrics may cause this to become worse. Later in life, when a child is moving about, the allergic reaction may be partly or solely caused by contact with substances touched, dust and animals especially. If you think your child may develop allergies, think very carefully before planning to have a pet.

About a third of infants who are atopic can expect to get eczema when given cow's milk, even if modified. That is, at least one in twenty of bottle-fed babies. Babies who are largely breast-fed halve the chance of developing eczema while those who only breast-feed reduce the risk to roughly one in a hundred. If breast-feeding is unsuccessful and needs to be replaced with bottle-feeding, do not be too concerned. Even breast-feeding for a few weeks or three months is remarkably effective in protecting a baby.

Cow's milk and eggs are almost always the chief culprits for eczema sufferers. It is wise to give these as late as possible and, if they do cause allergy, to exclude them from the diet. In a few cases quite dramatic results have occurred by changing to goat's or sheep's milk, so even if it gives only moderate help it is wise to try for a period of two to three months if your child has moderate or severe eczema. If your child is over one year, there is no need for medical approval. Breast-feed for at least one year if you can.

Eggs are not normally given until six months for the average child, but those at risk of developing eczema are advised to wait for one or even two years. If, when eggs are first offered, they are rejected, make a point of giving no more – even in a disguised form – for several months.

By eight to nine months, your baby should be able to eat many family foods, so long as they do not contain cow's milk or eggs. Plan meals to suit everyone as far as possible.

Eczema waxes and wanes for a variety of reasons other than diet: hot weather, the type of clothes worn, how tense or upset the child is, whether he is free of minor complaints like colds. To thus isolate what foods are causing allergies can be very difficult. It is usually wise to seek medical help and advice and as much information as possible from books. The Eczema Society in particular, will have the most up-to-date information, and they give local group support (see Appendix II).

Do remember to consult your doctor if you are using creams etc. on a child's skin for eczema *before* you plan to become pregnant again. Some medications are not suitable for skin contact with an expectant mother. Remember also to tell your doctor of allergies in the family, especially of an egg allergy, before your baby's immunisation programme begins. Children should not receive smallpox vaccine if they or another member of the family has eczema. Diptheria, whooping cough, tetanus (DPT) and polio *can* be given, as can German measles. But those allergic to eggs should not be given measles, flu or yellow fever inoculations.

Overweight in eczema sufferers may aggravate their condition, both as babies and children. Deeper creases at wrists, elbows, knees, etc. will cause these areas to irritate more, and chafing of the dry skin in overweight limbs may be painful, especially between the legs. Infants and children with a tendency to chubbiness should have their diet watched carefully, and every effort should be made to see good eating habits are established.

Additions to the diet
Research into eczema has shown abnormalities in the body's fatty acids, which have led to the recommendation that sunflower seed oil may be helpful in the diet – about 2 teaspoons a day – but start with ¼

Keep eczema at bay

1. Use chicken stock, not milk, for sauces for meat, fish, vegetables, or use soya or goat's milk.

2. Use kosher (Jewish) margarine or some of the slimmers' 'margarines' which contain no milk or whey.

3. Choose cereals without dried milk added. Avoid Special K and Coco-pops. Check contents of muesli, oat cereals and all other breakfast cereals. A wide range do not contain milk. Serve to eczema sufferers with goat or low-allergy milk.

4. Give fruit jellies, pies, tarts, crumbles, not sponge puddings containing eggs. Avoid mousses, ice cream, yogurt (except goat's milk yogurt).

5. Avoid lemon curd, chocolate, fudge toffee, salad cream and mayonnaise which often contain milk or eggs.

6. Avoid tinned and prepared meats, burgers, sausages, commercial pies and pasties, any of which may contain milk or egg. Tinned or packaged goods may list contents which can be checked. Local butchers will advise if their sausages or burgers are milk- or egg-free (explain why you are asking and they are sure to be helpful).

7. Choose brands of breads, biscuits and cakes that list contents you can check. Look out for whey, casein, lactose, which are derived from milk. Local bakeries can advise on all their products.

8. Coatings on fish may contain eggs or milk. Frozen products will list contents.

9. All baby foods contain precise lists of contents as do other tinned foods. When using these, check and choose carefully. Avoiding cow's milk and eggs until after twelve months is a precaution for those who have shown early signs of eczema.

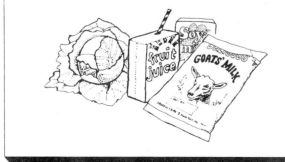

to ½ teaspoon from four to nine months, and build up gradually. This may improve the skin. Too much will cause overweight. Later in life, the use of sunflower seed or corn oil in preference to other oils for salads etc. may be sufficient without a measured dose. You could also add the oil to cereal, fruit or vegetable purées, etc., as you serve them. Do not give by the spoonful to young children – it will not be very acceptable.

Give plenty of vitamins too. Some sufferers find Vitamin C improves their skin; others Vitamin E or B (as brewer's yeast tablets). Others find black molasses, radishes or watercress help.

As wise and healthy a diet as is possible with a minimum of sugar should be aimed at by all eczema sufferers. Eat foods high in pantothenic acid (or the B vitamins): wheat or rice bran, wheatgerm, peanuts, sesame seed, pulses, eggs, offal or brewer's yeast tablets, plus yogurt daily if possible. Vitamin and mineral supplements should be added if allergies exclude important ingredients of the diet. This should be accompanied by a well ordered, calm life-style, and careful consideration of all other external factors which can affect the skin.

Asthma

During an asthma attack, the air passages in the lungs narrow, and this causes great difficulties in breathing. A baby or child becomes panicky and frightened, which makes the condition worse. One in twenty children suffer from asthma and of them two-thirds are boys. As babies, these children may have shown signs of eczema or had wheezing or bronchial conditions, and may develop asthma at about two years. All of these symptoms should be carefully studied to see if the cause can be removed. Fortunately, many children grow out of asthma at seven years and still more are clear by their mid-teens.

In many infants, diet is of less importance than external irritants such as dust, pollen, animals, cold winds, fumes, and members of the family smoking, so these should be given careful consideration. A fairly dust and pollution free environment, particularly at night, without smokers, animals and flowers in the house, should be encouraged. Tree pollen in April and May and grass pollen in June and July may make these the most difficult months of the year if pollens are a major cause. Care should also always be taken to avoid bed-making and vacuum-cleaning in the presence of an asthmatic child. Vigorous bread-making where flour grains are in the air may also be an irritant. Choose house plants for their leaves alone.

If a mother, father, or grandparent has eczema, a child may inherit sensitivity and could develop eczema, asthma or both. Similarly asthma may be passed down and eczema develop. As with eczema, breast-feeding has been shown to be a major protective factor, especially if great care is taken to avoid cow's milk.

The most usual foods linked to the incidence of asthma attacks are cow's milk and eggs, so complete avoidance of these for as long as possible is wise if your child is wheezy or at risk of being atopic. Nut milks (and nuts) are not recommended as some asthmatics are shown to be allergic to nuts. Soya milk, water or breast milk should be used when preparing rice cereal. Eggs alone will not often be the total cause, nor for that matter, cow's milk, but if partial relief is obtained by leaving them out, it will be worthwhile. Fish and chocolate may also trigger asthma attacks, so leave out for the wheezy baby and introduce with care after two years.

Vitamin A is needed for the good working of the mucous lining of the lungs and it is present in liver, carrots and dark green vegetables, apricots and peaches (also milk, butter, cheese, and eggs, of which the asthmatic child may be taking very little). Vitamin C will help protect the child from colds and other chest infections, which make the asthma worse, so it is wise to give the recommended dose of vitamin supplements until seven years of A, D and C plus the B vitamins to ensure the good health of your child.

Every effort should be made to ensure chesty children remain slim. This puts less strain on their lungs (and hearts), especially when taking exercise. It has also been shown that slim babies and children are less prone to colds and chest infections. Keep a careful record of your baby's or child's weight if they are inclined to be chubby and make sure high-calorie foods, especially those with little food value, are avoided or restricted. Serve fresh fruit regularly instead of cooked puddings. It is very tempting for a mother to comfort a suffering child with sweets, biscuits, cakes and pop, but these should be avoided in favour of healthier foods.

Further information concerning care and environment for an asthmatic can be obtained from the Asthma Research Council (see Appendix II).

Migraine

Migraine usually takes the form of unexpected severe headaches, and often the child vomits or feels very sick. Headaches that are associated with childhood infections – colds, flu etc. – are not migraine and have an obvious cause. Those in an otherwise healthy child may be migraine. In some children, especially younger children, there is no headache, just vomiting. This used to be called a bilious attack. Some children may only have recurrent unexplained tummy ache, which is sometimes diagnosed as a form of migraine. More typical migraine with headaches may not occur until after seven years, or later in the teens.

The most typical symptoms are: pain at one side of the head, often behind the eye; short period of disturbed vision, with light spots, black areas, or strange sensations like numbness, tingling, paralysis, or inability to speak, or slurred speech. Children's descriptions of these sensations may sound remarkably like *Alice in Wonderland*, a feeling of falling down holes, walking in tunnels, shrinking, or the walls closing in. Lewis Carroll was a migraine sufferer too, which explains why the symptoms sound familiar! Migraine normally runs in the family, so is often recognised by the fellow sufferer. Small children under seven, especially, may confuse the headache with earache or toothache. A feeling of shivering, yawning, pale face with dark rings round the eyes and sense of disorientation are the signs a mother may notice. Children can have a temperature with migraine; few do, and while the attack may last only an hour, it can last two to three days. Childhood migraine is believed to affect as many as 750,000 children under ten in the UK. It affects as many boys as girls to start with, but by seven years, many children, especially the boys, grow out of it, and by eleven to twelve years, still more have done so. About one in four women have a period of migraine at some time in their lives and about one in eight men.

Migraine is closely linked with food and eating habits. Stress and excitement play an important part, but often eating a particular food may be the final trigger of an attack. It is believed that there are many migraine sufferers who are unable to get rid of some types of amines present in food and that these build up in the blood to trigger an attack. Isolating which amines are the culprit and in which foods these are present might need the help of a dietician, but many of the common trigger foods are quickly spotted. One point to be remembered is that a trigger food may often be eaten with no ill effect, but at other times – when stressed or excited as at parties, school outings, exams – the food can cause an attack. Eating that food several times over a short period – citrus fruits in the winter for instance – can also cause a reaction.

Other migraine sufferers can have attacks, not

Less common migraine triggers

Some foods upset a comparatively smaller number of people and might be considered worth omitting for a short period, or at least carefully checking against a record of food eaten before previous attacks. These are:

- Milk, cream, butter and other dairy products.
- Yogurt. Like cheese it contains tyramine.
- Fried foods.
- Certain vegetables – onions and baked beans, for instance – contain tyramine.
- Some fruits other than citrus, especially ripe bananas, or unripe green apples.
- Pork is the meat most frequently associated with migraine; beef affects others.
- Tea and coffee.
- Yeast and Marmite (contain tyramine).
- Fish, particularly shellfish.
- Sugar, or a sudden high intake of sweet foods, as at tea parties and afternoon teas.
- Salt, particularly when sprinkled on food like crisps, peanuts, chips and eaten on an empty stomach late in the day. (Normal salt content is not suspect).

because of what they consume, but because they have gone too long without food or drink. Few sufferers are sufficiently aware of this or conscious of the gap between meals and so frequently blame a particular food quite incorrectly.

When children have an attack of migraine, it is wise to write up a record on not only what they have eaten in the previous twenty-four hours, but of *when* they ate. In addition to this a record of activities – party, late night, late lie-in, sports, school outing – is useful as these may not only affect the times meals were taken, but vigorous activities will increase the need for food, so a shorter gap between meals may be necessary. A comparison of three or four of these recorded attacks may enable you to easily pinpoint the problem for yourself. Random questions from a doctor about past attacks are unlikely to reveal the cause so clearly, and memory is often faulty about previous occasions, especially regarding times of meals. His help in prescribing special drugs when aspirin is insufficient is of course invaluable. Your record of intake may be most helpful to him, if isolating a problem food is proving difficult.

There are four very common foods which affect migraine sufferers: chocolate, cheese, citrus fruits, and alcohol (which last, of course, is irrelevant for children). A specific amine, tyramine, has been isolated as one major cause.

Those suffering from migraine would be wise to omit chocolate (and cocoa), cheese (and usually yogurt) and citrus fruits completely from their diet for a period of one to two months to see if this in any way lessens their attacks. Three-quarters of migraine sufferers find chocolate does not suit them and nearly half are upset by cheese. Around a third react to citrus fruits. This is especially common when taken at breakfast or on an empty stomach.

It is not recommended that a diet excluding all the less common trigger foods (see left) should be tried. Most people are only upset by a small number of foods and records taken before previous attacks should easily narrow down suspect foods. Certain smells may also trigger an attack of migraine – raw leek, onion, alcohol, vinegar, peppermint, etc.

Food which may help

Honey is one food many sufferers claim to be a great help. It is therefore possibly a wise choice at breakfast, instead of marmalade (containing citrus fruits) or Marmite, which may be a trigger also.

A diet rich in wheat bran, wholemeal bread, whole-grain breakfast cereals, rice, pasta and plenty of dietary fibre in other ways is recommended. Migraine sufferers are often constipated at the time of an attack, although whether the constipation causes migraine or vice-versa is unclear.

Drinking water from the tap or bottled spa water is definitely good for all, but especially migraine sufferers. Large quantities of coffee or tea, milk or citrus juices rarely suit them so small children should acquire the habit of drinking 1 pint (575 ml) water a day, and adults up to 2½ pints (1.4 litres). Many children are allowed to drink quantities of squash and pop which are not as suitable for the body as plain water for flushing out body waste.

Feverfew (*pyrethrum parthenium*), is a plant grown easily in England. It has been classed as a medicinal herb for many centuries and was traditionally used in the treatment of fevers and headaches. Available in health-food shops dried, it is not recommended in pregnancy and *not* for young children until further tested.

Feeding migraine sufferers

Many mothers do not notice the long gaps their children go without food. We are used to babies being fed roughly every four hours, but many children and adults should not be allowed to go more than four to five hours without food, or a maximum of thirteen hours at night. Longer than this will, in some, trigger migraine attacks. This obviously means planning a day with three main meals and two to three small snacks. These last do not need to be large – a suitable drink may be enough – possibly with plain biscuit, toast or fruit.

When there is a weekend late lie-in followed by a late family breakfast, it is wise to give young children cereals at their normal breakfast time at least, even if a cooked breakfast is served much later.

At most nursery schools, children are expected to have mid-morning nourishment. In junior school, those prone to headaches in the morning would be wise to have some suitable snack. This is particularly important for many children at times of school outings, say, when lunchtime may be delayed.

Migraine sufferers are usually fitter if they have a hot meal at midday, not a cold lunch. School lunches may seem preferable to packed lunch, but the benefit will be lost if the child does not eat the food because it is unsuitable (cheese and onion pie, fried fish and chips and chocolate puddings) or not liked and, as a result, the child goes hungry for too long. Packed hot lunches are not difficult to arrange. An unbreakable thermos can be used (see packed lunches, Chapter Six). On return from school, children should be given food and drink as soon as possible, especially after sporting activities, when calories will have been used up more quickly.

In some children, a bad alignment of teeth may cause pressure in the jaw and result in teeth-grinding and possibly migraine headaches. If children grind their teeth at night, arrange a dental check. Chewing food may appear to trigger migraine, but for the health of the teeth and jaw plenty of foods should be given which require chewing. Nevertheless, at the onset of an attack, a migraine sufferer may find eating softer foods a better choice. If children return from school with the beginning of a headache and can be persuaded to take hot food such as soup, Bovril with bread dunked in, or other hot food requiring little chewing, this may arrest the attack. Milk drinks are less likely to be suitable, so are cold and fizzy drinks.

Making sure migraine sufferers have something to eat and drink *before* going to a party will ensure that they are not too exhausted, thirsty and hungry at tea-time and can enjoy the party tea, and avoid, if they themselves wish, any suspect trigger foods. Iced drinks and iced foods can be a trigger to some children, especially when hot after lively games.

For further information and advice concerning migraine, plus support groups contact the Migraine Trust (see Appendix II).

Hyperactivity

This condition is not recognised by all doctors, but is beginning to attract greater concern and interest.

Infants and children are described as hyperactive if they seem in a perpetual state of motion, highly excitable and fretful, often with poor coordination in movement or speech. They have poor concentration, although they may be of normal or above average intelligence. These children sleep badly, are thirsty and many have other known allergic problems, like asthma, hayfever, headaches and catarrh. The symptoms may sound like the lively mischievous behaviour of most three-year-olds, but the degree of anti-social behaviour is such that they are very difficult to integrate in playgroups as toddlers or take to any public place without causing scenes. As fretful babies, they may cause baby battering if the mother (or father) is not given sufficient family and medical support. As infants, they often indulge in cot-rocking, head-banging, or other obsessive habits, although these alone do not indicate that a child is or will become hyperactive.

It is now widely recognised that high lead levels in the blood can cause brain damage and anti-social behaviour in young children and teenagers. Lead may be present in canned food (tins are sealed with lead), oily fish, and in many foods grown in urban areas. But the prime source in many is inhalation of petrol exhaust fumes, and dust from old paintwork or urban environments. Cadmium and other heavy metals are also suspect. All fruit and vegetables should be washed before preparation to ensure any external contamination is removed, and all children trained to wash their hands before handling food or putting fingers in their mouths.

There appear to be some children whose behaviour and health becomes abnormal when they eat particular 'foods'. Those items which are most suspect are the synthetic chemical additives such as synthetic food colouring and nitrates and nitrites (used in the preparation of bacon, ham, other cured meats, sausages and cheese); monosodium glutamate and synthetic flavourings as well as some antioxidants.

Children who are hyperactive may also be allergic to salicylates in their diet. This chemical, present in aspirin, occurs naturally in most fruits including all berries, currants, apples, oranges, tomatoes and cucumber, but excluding lemon, grapefruit, banana, pear, pineapple, melon and avocado. Children may be advised to avoid all artificial additives plus fruits containing salicylates for four to six weeks, then if health is improved return the fruits gradually to the diet, so long as no poor reaction occurs. Many medicaments – toothpaste and vitamin supplements for children and infants – contain artificial food colour, flavour or salicylates. Your doctor can prescribe medicaments free of these and a chemist will point out suitable vitamin supplements; always choose uncoloured toothpaste. What has been noticed about most hyperactive children is that there are nine times as many boys affected as girls, and it is more common when parents smoke. The affected children are often extremely thirsty and many have an unusually low level of the mineral zinc.

Babies and children who appear hyperactive should be seen by their doctor so that he can check for such causes as lead poisoning, hypoglycaemia, specific allergies or digestive disorders. If the infant or child shows no specific problem, mothers will find much comfort and support by contacting other mothers who have gone through a similarly distressing period with their own child. Excluding food additives from the diet and processed foods in favour of wholemeal bread, uncured meats – beef, lamb, pork and poultry – and a wide range of vegetables, both green and pulses, may be helpful. Avoiding fruits containing salicylates is only worthwhile if a strict diet excluding added chemicals is being followed. These fruits should only be kept out of the diet if there is an obvious benefit to the infant. All lively infants and children have high nutritional requirements to maintain good health. They need more than average B, C, D and E vitamins, calcium, magnesium and zinc. A good diet with plenty of fresh milk, yeast extract, liver and wheatgerm, plus vitamin supplements will supply this, but a diet high in white flour, sugar, sweets, soft drinks and pop should be avoided at all costs to prevent the energetic child becoming fractious and disruptive.

Detailed information on suitable foods for the hyperactive child as well as local support groups can be provided by the Hyperactive Children's Support Group (see Appendix II), and the Feingold diet used as the basis of their recommendations may be useful for some sufferers of eczema, asthma and migraine.

Skin rashes

Urticaria, or nettle-rash as it is often called, is a fairly common reaction to some foods, particularly strawberries, shellfish, eggs and nuts, as well as some drugs. It can also be caused by touching certain garden and house plants, or hairy caterpillars, and it may spread from the hands to the face, neck and body.

Contact dermatitis

Avoid biological washing machine powders (Ariel) and anti-bacterial soaps (Shield). The commonest contact dermatitis in babies is nappy rash. Use 1 to 2 tablespoons of vinegar in the final rinse of the nappies, as well as protective creams and nappy liners. Rash in the nappy area may also have been caused by a food to which there is an allergy, if simple precautions – like cleanliness and cream – have not been effective.

Allergic catarrh

Infants and children with permanently runny noses can be suspected of an allergic catarrh and the cause should be sought by checking whether the child is allergic to milk or eggs, or some other food, or whether it is inhaled substances which are the primary cause.

Croup

Usually due to an infection, but can be brought on by an allergic reaction. A third cause may be the result of inhaling an object, when, for instance, food may have got into the lungs. Any child with breathing difficulties should be seen promptly by a doctor. Advise him if you suspect choking – especially on a peanut.

Allergic stomach upset

A bloated uncomfortable feeling in the stomach may be due to an allergic condition. Improper digestion of food may cause gas to be formed. Alternatively there may be diarrhoea, vomiting or just pain. A tummy bug or food poisoning could be the cause, but if a child suffers from regular, frequent or continuous stomach upsets, an allergy is more probable. A record of food eaten in the previous few meals should be noted and discussed with a doctor. Stomach upsets may also involve emotional factors, as in migraine.

Coeliac disease

A digestive disorder which is similar and possibly linked to allergies. In coeliac disease, the lining of the small intestine is damaged when gliadin (part of the protein gluten) is consumed, which affects the intestine's ability to absorb other foods and the infant, in addition to showing upset bowels (as fatty diarrhoea), will lose weight and become malnourished. Gliadin occurs in the gluten of wheat and rye and also in barley and oats. To ensure that all infants have the best possible health in the first months of life, these cereals should be omitted from the diet until six to seven months in favour of rice (or maize) cereal. Any child who develops persistent diarrhoea, a pot belly and loses weight after mixed cereals are introduced, should therefore be checked and monitored by the doctor.

Coeliac disease has a slight tendency to run in families. About one in 1,500 are diagnosed in the UK, but in the West of Ireland this may be as high as one in 300. In negroes and orientals it is almost unknown. Sufferers are more prone to allergic complaints such as eczema, migraine, etc. than average. Too early an introduction to foods containing gluten is not a prime cause, but allowing the potential sufferer to develop for six to seven months without risk of upset is obviously better than a much smaller baby being exposed to a debilitating disease.

A coeliac's diet can be low in dietary fibre with whole-wheat products omitted. This should be made up for by using whole-grain brown rice and pulse vegetables – lentils, haricot beans, etc. – regularly, also by serving potatoes cooked in their skins and a good range of salads, green vegetables and fruits. A jacket potato with cheese or other topping or home-made vegetable soup, plus fruit and yogurt, makes a good tea-time choice for children, when sandwiches, cakes, biscuits might otherwise have been served. Dried fruit makes a good snack as an alternative to biscuits. For making home-made shortbread and similar biscuits, gluten-free flour and one-third ground rice or cornflour can replace the ordinary flour. Fruit cakes and whisked sponge cakes are also successful using gluten-free flour.

All those medically diagnosed as suffering from coeliac disease can obtain an annually up-dated list of gluten-free manufactured products by joining the Coeliac Society. Baby foods are now being marked with the crossed grain (see page 54) if gluten-free, but most manufactured foods for children and adults will give no indication and special lists are needed. Chemists and health-food shops may stock specially prepared gluten-free flour for home cooking. By getting in touch with a local group of sufferers, you may jointly persuade local bakers to make occasional batches of gluten-free bread and butchers, gluten-free sausages or burgers, which can be bought in bulk to freeze.

Some items may be available on prescription. Check with your doctor or health visitor for what is currently available. The address of the Coeliac Society is available from your doctor when the disease is diagnosed.

Chapter Ten
What else do parents need to know?

Travelling with babies and children

It is surprising how flexible both mother and baby and children can be when travelling. If you are planning a holiday with a long journey, it is a good idea to do a few day-trips first as practice. Do not set off armed to the teeth for every eventuality where food and drinks are concerned, but learn to use what you find to some extent. You may find the following advice particularly helpful if travelling abroad.

Babies' milk feeds

Finding suitable places to feed your baby away from home is much easier than it used to be. Most people are much more accustomed to seeing babies bottle- or breast-fed in more public places. Ladies' waiting rooms and cloakrooms in stores often have a suitable place where a mother may breast-feed. Carry a fashionable shawl to throw over your shoulder if you wish to discreetly feed your baby on buses, taxis or planes, in the car or in restaurants.

For bottle-feeding, take with you boiled water either hot in a thermos or cold in feeding bottles. If baby is under seven to eight months take suitable dried baby milk with you. It is often safer not to change brands when on holiday so take as much as you will probably need. If you are in transit and cannot sterilise bottle properly in containers, when you have used bottle wash in tap water, then fill with water adding a quarter sterilising tablet; insert teat upside down, seal and then screw on top.

Over seven months babies can be given any dried milk for an occasional feed in an emergency, but it is much better to use evaporated milk or UHT milk from cartons, or bottled sterilised milk for everyday use. Do *not* use chocolate or other flavoured milks. Dried milks – either modified baby milk or those suitable for older consumption – are the most convenient for mixing while in transit since dry products will not deteriorate until reconstituted.

When you arrive at your destination, especially if abroad, evaporated milk is a good choice for older babies (seven months plus) and young children. Use it occasionally before you go so they get used to the taste. It is of a good standard and widely available throughout the world; you do not need to travel with a case full. Store opened can in refrigerator and use within forty-eight hours, and dilute as you use (one part evaporated milk to one and a half parts water: in USA, one to one – just in case the instructions are in Arabic!). Unopened tins can be kept anywhere, and do remember to wipe the tops well first.

Try to accustom baby to taking milk cold if you can, it makes life easier. Nevertheless planes and restaurants should be able to heat a bottle for you and waiting rooms, cloakrooms and trains usually have hot running water with which you can take the chill off a cold bottle.

Babies' solid food

Most of the following – if not exactly gastronomic – should ensure baby is well fed! For small babies of four to seven months the dried packet foods are a useful standby for many meals (one main meal a day). If going abroad take some packets with you and check with travel agent on available items. Most tourist centres in Europe have excellent baby food available in jars or dried – some are superior to British brands – so you will not need to take a case full.

Cereals
Dry cereals to mix with milk or formula are very convenient to transport, but are also available quite

readily abroad. If you are self-catering any local grains may be cooked as a porridge; if in an hotel bread may be soaked in milk as a cereal in an emergency.

Fruits

Bananas are widely available and a perfect easy food at four to six months; other fruit, ripe and washed, can be given raw. Fruit and salads are best washed in bottle sterilising solution in Mediterranean countries. You do not need special equipment or a bowl; cut in half or cut out slices according to size. Remove any seeds, pips or stones. Scrape fruit flesh to pulp using teaspoon as you feed baby holding fruit in skin. Discard any left over in this skin. Wrap up portion of fruit not used for next meal if wished.

Tinned fruits can also be used. Discard sweet syrup and use small hand food-mill or mash with fork. Plain apple sauce in tins and jars may be available, but avoid pie fillings.

Vegetables

Mashed potato is excellent but avoid instant mash as it is high in additives and lower in food value.

Carrots and cucumber are good finger foods – continental cucumber is rather bitter. Cooked carrots and peas can be mashed. Tinned baked beans can be used occasionally at seven to eight months, then regularly after that. Other tinned beans and peas should have liquid drained off, and if salted, mash with milk or water.

Eggs and yogurt, etc

Boiled eggs are very portable; the yolks can be soft or hard-cooked and can be easily ordered at restaurants. Mash and fruit juice, milk or yogurt.

Caramel or plain egg custards are usually on the menu. Do not serve the sweet caramel sauce. You will be able to purchase yogurt; use from cartons, not open bowls, for safety. Choose plain yogurt and check the list of contents on fruit flavoured; do not buy chocolate or coffee flavours, and check nut yogurts are not too coarse for babies.

Meat

Tinned spreads and tinned pâtés are high in additives but could be used very occasionally with vegetable purée.

Tinned meats – mince, spaghetti with meatballs, stews, chicken and also macaroni cheese – can be used occasionally. Check list of contents; most are high in salt so it's not wise to use under eight months. Toddlers and young children can be given tinned sardines, mackerel and tuna.

Cheese

Cottage cheese and Petit Suisse are low fat and can be fed to baby. Mash with fork if too coarse, adding extra milk, fruit juice or fruit purée. Check list of contents and date stamp on carton. Older children can be given a wide range of cheese with local fresh bread for a quick easy meal.

Continental dishes

Mediterranean people are much more tolerant of babies and children in public places and restaurants and take delight in making you feel at home with them generally. They do not share the prevalent UK attitude that children should be seen and not heard. Children will be welcome in restaurants and so long as staff are not too busy they will often be most helpful if you want jugs of hot water to heat bottles. Try to be self-sufficient as much as possible for your own peace of mind, or make sure you arrive early before the crowd if you want preferential treatment.

Sensible Continental choices

Italy
Vegetable soups. Add Parmesan cheese.
Pasta. Spaghetti Bolognese, Lasagne, Cannelloni etc.
Risotto, Polenta, Casseroles and Sautés (of chicken, lamb, liver and white fish).

France
Pilaff, Risotto.
Soups, Ragoûts, Sautés and Casseroles (of meat and white fish).

Spain
Rice dishes and **Paella** (without shellfish).
Casseroles, Sautés (of chicken, lamb, liver, white fish) and **Omelettes**.

Ice creams

Always popular on holiday, but only buy wrapped ices or those from dispensing machines. *Do not* buy ice cream doled out in scoops. The jug of tepid water used for storing scoops must be an ideal breeding ground for bacteria.

Choose vanilla ice cream first then fruit ice creams. Sorbets, water ices and ice lollies have little or no nutritional value while dairy ices contain protein, fat and calcium. Do not give a baby chocolate or nut ice creams. Watch the quantity of ice cream children eat, and cut out sweets and biscuits altogether if they are having more than one or two a day.

Many toddlers and young children are highly conservative on holiday. Do not worry if their diet is not very varied for this short period. If they only eat omelette, a burger and chips every day plus ice cream, try to balance this with plenty of fresh fruit – about three fruits a day. Bread and cheese makes an easy picnic lunch for all over two and by this age bought pâté and cold meats are suitable. A large choice is available all over the Continent, but choose tinned or vacuum packed if you are worried about local hygiene standards.

Cereals at breakfast usually help ensure a good milk intake so are no bad routine to continue even abroad. Cornflakes and Rice Krispies are available in many countries. Packets of ProNutro or Ready-brek do not take up much room so take them with you, and ask the staff to supply hot or cold milk to mix with them.

Drinks

Apart from milk drinks, good fruit juices can easily be bought. To make more refreshing dilute with water. Bottled water or 'Sterotabs' should be used if local water is not considered safe. It is wise to use one of these along the Mediterranean coasts as northern visitors may not be immune to the local bacteria. Pop is usually considered safe from bacteria, although normally not really advisable for young (or older) children: 7-Up or Sprite have the least chemical additives.

Do not add ice to any drinks when abroad. Chilled liquid inactivates the stomach's defence mechanism to bacteria, and the ice will have been made from untreated water. This is most important for children and good advice for adults in a hot climate – although it may mean going without the holiday delight of cocktails on the rocks!

Flying with baby and young children

You may be stuck longer than you expect at airports through flight delays. Carry adequate milk for baby, drinks for children, and fruit, yogurts or sandwiches for snacks. Airport food can be very expensive and often it is limited in choice – with chocolate cake and no fresh fruit, for instance – or your young child may not like the food supplied (on the whole this has gradually been much improved).

Ensure when the plane descends that a baby is able to suck at breast or bottle to release any painful pressure on the ears. This is one of the rare times when sucking boiled sweets or peppermints can be recommended for children!

Travelling by car, bus and train

Children find eating helps break up a tedious journey but it can be extremely messy. Those over seven can usually manage to drink from a small screw-top bottle if the family want to save unnecessary stops. Smaller children need more careful supervision, and cups with sucking spouts may be better for them. Store in poly bag or box. Plan ahead and choose non messy food to take.

- Small pots and bags of dried fruit.
- Apples, bananas.
- Small firm sandwiches. Wrap individually in foil or film to hand out.
- Sticks of celery, carrots and cucumber in bag or box.
- Fingers of cheese and cold sausages (wrap end in foil to hold).
- Plain biscuits or crackers.
- A cooler bag will help keep food fresh longer, and do not forget a damp cloth or pre-moistened wipes.

Poisons

Poisoning accidents happen even in the most conscientious households so parents should never feel so ashamed of their negligence that they are embarrassed to seek medical help. If you believe your child has taken a poisonous substance always act promptly and do not wait to see if he or she develops any symptoms. Ring your doctor if in any doubt, and if away from home, ring the emergency services, call at the nearest hospital, or even at a chemist's for advice.

The peak time for accidents is around 8 to 9 in the morning, according to statistics. A horrifying 80 per cent of poisoning accidents involve under-fives; most are between eighteen and thirty-six months. Aspirin causes about 25 per cent of accidents; 50 per cent are caused by other tablets (including the birth pill); and the remaining 25 per cent are due to poisoning by household and garden products, plants and seeds.

Times of greatest risk

1. When one member of the family is ill and the medicine cupboard is in regular use. Tablets may be left in a patient's room (an adult invalid may fall asleep and not notice a child slip into the room).

2. When you have guests staying. Many older adults may have forgotten what small children can get up to and leave sleeping tablets etc., by the bed. Teenage and many adult visitors have little conception of the danger of leaving aspirins etc. around in a household with toddlers.

3. When you are visiting friends and relatives. Their homes may not be designed for the protection of youngsters once children have grown past the dangerous age (over seven to nine years old), or have not yet reached mobility. Families are usually very casual about leaving aspirins on kitchen shelves and a variety of poisons under the kitchen sink. Take a roll of sticky tape with you to seal cupboards and drawers.

4. When you are setting off on holiday. When you are getting out holiday medicaments and preoccupied with arrangements, it is very easy not to transfer items straight from a locked cupboard to a locked suitcase.

5. When you are on holiday. Remember to keep medicaments in a locked suitcase and return them promptly when used.

6. When you are spring-cleaning, turning out cupboards, drawers etc.

7. When parents are arguing.

8. When shopping. Do not put small child in back of car with basket of shopping beside him or place unsuitable shopping items in or on a pram.

9. When you are busy at breakfast time or bathing baby. Make sure you have not left poisons around.

Poisons in the house and garden

Major dangers in the kitchen
Washing-up liquid, detergents, soap powders and mild disinfectants are not likely to put a child's life at risk, but store with care. Keep range of cleaning materials to a minimum for easier safe storage. The greatest risks of very dangerous poisoning are from the following:

Dishwasher Powder Store on very high shelf or locked cupboard.

Metal Polishes Buy only impregnated wadding cleansers while children are young.

Dry Cleaning Fluids Use only those with padded top (Dabitoff), not bottles of liquid paraffin or meths which are highly dangerous. Keep locked away.

Kettle Descalers Avoid using and having in the house if possible, as they are *very* dangerous.

Bleach Keep locked away, toddlers can quickly drink a lethal quantity.

Iron Tablets Very dangerous, so store with the greatest caution, as many look very tempting to toddlers. Vitamin drops are better than vitamin supplements that tend to look like mini-Smarties. Choose drops for Vitamins A and D until the youngest member of the family is over four.

Major dangers in the bathroom
Make sure you have a child-proof cupboard.

Sedatives and Sleeping Tablets Flush away any no longer in regular use. Be *very* cautious as side effects may make their user less able to judge whether they are safely locked away.

Camphor or Camphorated Oil Do not keep in house with young children.

Perfumes, Special Medicated Shampoos and Acne Preparations Keep them all in locked cupboard. Other make-up is harmless.

Cough Mixtures Do not leave in child's bedroom when ill. Return to locked cupboard.

Major dangers in garden and garage
Use powder and granular chemicals, not liquids. Do not store in diluted form. Keep garden chemicals to an absolute minimum for safety. Store all in a locked cupboard.

Paraquat or Liquid Dinitro-ortho-cresol Do not use. Buy only essential weed killers from chemist and ask advice of trained chemist on safety with young children if in any doubt.

Petrol and Fuel Keep in locked cupboards.

Emergency action in cases of poisoning

It is sometimes necessary to induce vomiting if a poison has been taken, especially for pills and plants. Do not give salt water or mustard. The best method is to put a finger at the back of a child's throat. If this proves difficult or unsuccessful, take the child promptly to your nearest hospital casualty department, or you could ring your doctor immediately for advice on emergency treatment.

Aspirin, Disprin, Codeine, Paracetamol Tablets

Toxic dose 12 months 1–2 tablets
2 years + 4–10 tablets
Do not wait for symptoms if you suspect these may have been swallowed. Act promptly, **induce vomiting**, and ring your doctor immediately. Take remaining pills with you to casualty department or clinic.

Acids (strong), Kettle Descalers

These will cause immediate burns to skin or mouth; they are extremely dangerous and highly acid. Wash off skin, and give milk to drink; **do not induce vomiting**, and take straight to nearest casualty department. Take acid to hospital, or note brand name and type and size of container.

Alkalis (strong), Paint Stripper, Bleach, Dish Washer Powder, Oven Cleaner

Symptoms may not occur for several minutes. Skin will feel soapy and then there will be very severe pain. Wash skin with neat vinegar, or acid substance (citric acid, cream of tartar, orange juice). Give plenty of real orange juice to drink or one part vinegar to ten parts water or squash, followed by several tablespoons of salad oil or plenty of milk. **Do not induce vomiting**. Take straight to casualty department. Take alkalis with you or note brand name, type and size.

Alcohol

Do not allow small children sips of alcohol. When your back is turned, especially at parties, they may go round finishing off drinks. Toddlers usually like the taste of beer and sweet sherry especially. Small quantities of wine, cider or beer will do little harm but spirits and stronger drinks will. Give lots of sweet liquids immediately if a little is taken. If a lot is taken or if child becomes very drowsy, contact your doctor immediately or take straight to hospital.

Antibiotics, Antihistamines

Induce vomiting, and contact doctor immediately.

Antidepressant Tablets, Sleeping Tablets, Sedatives

Take straight to casualty department with remaining medication.

Antiseptics

Check containers. Some will say 'External Use Only' and are poisonous; others are not highly toxic. Contact doctor for advice, naming brand and type.

Camphor and Camphorated Oil

Act fast and take to casualty department.

Carbon Tetrachloride (dry-cleaning fluid), Meths, Petrol, Paraffin, Turps, Perfume

Fresh air. Contact doctor immediately. **Do not induce vomiting.**

Detergents, Upholstery, Carpet and Hair Shampoos

Give plenty of milk. **Induce vomiting** if more than 1 tablespoon consumed. For special medicated shampoo contact doctor for advice.

Disinfectants

Mild varieties like pine are harmless in small quantities. Seek medical advice if large amount taken or if in any doubt. For strong disinfectants, give plenty of milk whisked with egg white, and take to casualty department.

Hair Dyes

Give milk and take to hospital.

Iron Tablets

Act very fast. **Induce vomiting** and take to nearest hospital immediately. From four to six tablets will cause severe symptoms; fourteen can be fatal.

Lavatory Cleansers (acid)

Never mix with bleach, or a chlorine gas produced could cause fatalities. Seek doctor's advice if any burns in or around mouth. Give milk.

Laxatives

Give anti-diarrhoea mixture in normal dose and if only a few or little taken. If large quantity consumed, **induce vomiting** first. Contact doctor if tummy pain severe.

Nappy Rinses

Dissolve little normal soap in water, add squash to act as antidote, and follow with plenty of milk.

The Pill

Induce vomiting if more than two to four weeks' supply taken.

Poisonous Plants

Fatalities from plant poisoning are extremely rare, as most plants classed as poisonous have to be eaten in fairly large quantities (more than 1 tablespoon) to be very dangerous. **Induce vomiting** if poisonous plants have been eaten, and rub cooking oil or butter in mouth if burning and give ice cream or ice lollies or cubes to suck. Take child to casualty department or ring doctor if highly toxic plant taken – red or black berries, lily of the valley, lupin, toadstools – and take plant seeds or leaves with you for identification.

Swallowed Objects

Coins and toys are not made of toxic metals. If something is swallowed, give child a normal diet without laxatives or other medications. You can give him bread, a bran cereal or baked beans so that the offending object has a well-padded journey through the body (most items will pass through harmlessly in under five days). If your child has stomach pains within the next two weeks, contact your doctor and advise him of the accident: he may wish to arrange an X-ray, or check your child in case an obstruction has occurred.

If a *sharp pointed or long object* is swallowed, ring doctor for advice immediately.

Weed Killers and Poisonous Garden Chemicals

Paraquat and dinitro-ortho-cresol are highly toxic. For all chemicals, follow instructions for use carefully. In case of accident ring doctor or hospital immediately for correct advice. They can check their updated list of different types and brands and tell you what treatment is needed. Prompt antidotes or stomach wash will be required for some but not all. Do not wait for symptoms.

Quick guide to poisoning action

Unconscious Patient

Do *not* give drink or induce vomiting.

If breathing
Lie in recovery position.

If not breathing
Give kiss of life.

Ask for medical aid. Indicate poison.
Patient should not be left unattended.

Conscious Patient

Corrosive acids and alkalis, plus
Which will cause burning on
tongue and lips.

OR

Petrol and spirit-based fluids
Will smell on breath.

Non-corrosive
All tablets, medicines plants.

Ask for medical aid. Indicate poison.

Do *not* induce vomiting.

Induce vomiting.

Give drink slowly to dilute poison.

Food poisoning

This *can* occur, even in the most immaculate home, but often is caused by bacterial contamination in commercial processes or at the shop. Meticulous hygiene and correct storage are the major things.

1. Buy food from good sources only.
2. Store cooked and raw foods well apart.
3. Cool food quickly and store in refrigerator.
4. Thaw frozen food properly before cooking or allow plenty of cooking time.
5. Scrub wooden boards and all working surfaces well, especially after handling raw chicken, meat and fish. Wipe down with hyperchlorite (bottle sterilising solution) or bleach.
6. Return ice cream and similar frozen products quickly to deep freeze. Choose soft scoop ices in preference to those that have to be half thawed before ices are scooped out.
7. Always sterilise baby's bottles and wash his equipment first.
8. Never allow pets around at meal times. Wash all their items well away from family equipment.

Foods at risk

Tinned goods
Most cases of food poisoning are caused by meat and fish processed abroad. Always throw out any tins with bulging ends, which spurt liquid, with traces of mould or an unexpected smell. If in doubt never taste to test – throw out.

Vacuum jars
Home bottling or canning of non-acid vegetables, meat and fish is not recommended for amateurs. Tomatoes and fruit are acid, thus easy and safe for the home cook to prepare with slow preservation methods. Commercial products with vacuum lids should make a 'pop' on opening.

Vegetables
Discard all green potatoes and cut off sprouted parts. Do not serve soaked dried kidney beans without thoroughly boiling (for at least 15 minutes).

Poultry
Almost 50 per cent of all chicken contains traces of salmonella. Always thaw thoroughly and cook properly. Pour on boiling liquid or fry to brown before using slow cooker. A stuffed chicken needs to be cooked longer to ensure heat is distributed right to the centre.

Meat and fish
Never buy cooked meats and fish that are stored on the same counter as raw. Cooked products should always be lifted with a special set of tongs only. Do not store cooked and raw side by side in the fridge, or allow liquid to drip from raw meat on to cooked products.

Fruit
Do not crack fruit stones and use kernels. A few apricot kernels are safe in jam but they, plus peach, cherry, plum and prune kernels, contain arsenic. Inadvertently swallowed whole stones like cherry are harmless but should not be encouraged. Remove all stones from fruit for children under four.

Drug dependence

Many parents imagine that their children will not be faced with this problem before their teens, but this is not so. By seven to eight, some children will be developing addictions or dependence on drugs.

Nicotine
Many children start smoking before eleven years. It causes addiction, damaging heart and lungs, so watch for signs of smell on breath or clothes.

Inhalants
Glue solvents, aerosol sprays, metal polish etc. cause brain damage and permanent damage to liver and kidneys. Mild inhalation will cause only euphoria but children may go on to take more which can be fatal. Store all these items in a safe place and be aware of possible misuse. Watch for abnormally dilated eyes, glazed expressions and excitability.

Caffeine
In coffee, tea and cola drinks, this causes restlessness and sleeplessness and, in extremes, strain on the heart. Do not allow children to drink quantities of these: not more than one to three cups (depending on age) at three spaced intervals per day (effect lasts up to four hours). Provide non-cola drinks at parties like Sprite, 7-Up, fizzy lemonade, orangeade etc. Drinking large quantities can cause dependence.

A craving for caffeine is not often a serious problem, but the use, even occasional use, of nicotine and inhalants are a real danger to health. All forms of dependency in a young child may lead to higher risk of dependence on stronger drugs later, and should be taken seriously.

Appendix One
Growth and weight gain

The growth and weight charts indicate the average size and weight of children and shows their expectations in teenage as well; 3 per cent can expect to be both outside the top and bottom limits. There is no cause for concern if these children can expect to inherit a larger or smaller frame than most. Those children who are above or below the weight limit, yet of a very average size, should be checked to ensure they are not over- or underweight and are in good health. Where the family is of a normal height they should also be checked by the doctor if their height is unusual.

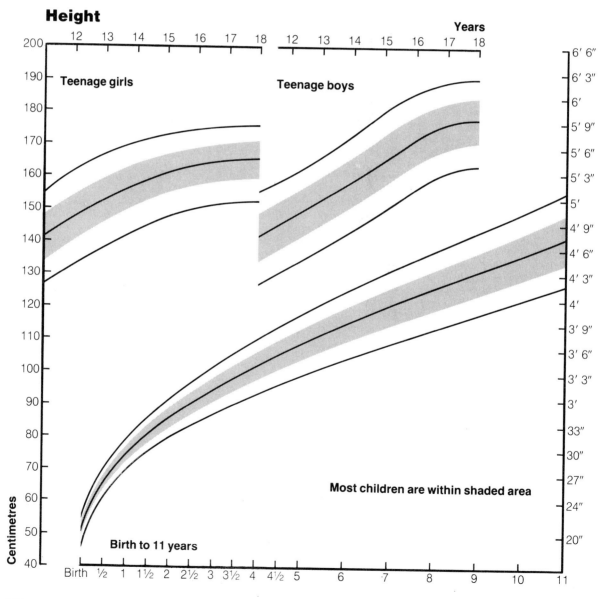

Height

Teenage girls

Teenage boys

Years

Most children are within shaded area

Birth to 11 years

Centimetres

Weight tends to continue to increase for boys after eighteen but steadies for girls around seventeen.

Growth and weight gain is not a steady process week by week but tends to go in leaps whether one is considering babies or older children.

As far as babies are concerned, between four and a half and five months the birth weight is expected to double. This is only one aspect of your baby's progress that will be checked at a baby clinic. After four to five months weight increase will slow down so that at twelve months all children may expect to be roughly three times their birth weight. Baby's length will increase by about 50 per cent – those 20 inches

(50 cm) long at birth can expect to be around 30 inches (75 cm) at twelve months.

Growth is at its slowest between one and a half and five to six years when appetite may appear small.

Boys and girls do not vary much until about nine to ten years when the girls begin their major growth spurt which tails off at fourteen to fifteen years. Boys start their growth spurt at around twelve to thirteen and by thirteen to fourteen years they will out-grow the girls, who are then nearly full grown, and will continue to grow about three years after the girls, to reach their adult height at around seventeen or eighteen.

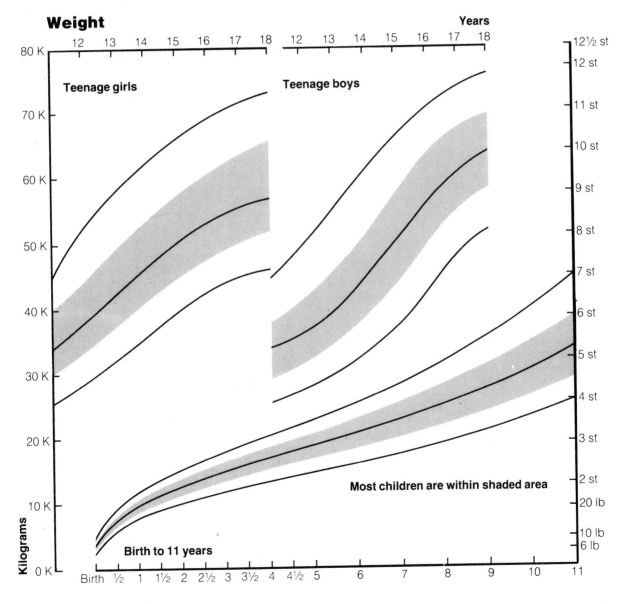

Appendix Two
Helpful organisations

Asthma
Asthma Research Council, 12 Pembridge Square, London W2 4EH

Before Conception
Foresight, The Old Vicarage, Church Lane, Witley, Godalming, Surrey, GU8 5PN

Breast-feeding
La Lèche League of Great Britain, Box 2424, London WC1X 6XX
The National Childbirth Trust, 9 Queensborough Terrace, London W2

Cot Deaths
Foundation for the Study of Infant Deaths (Cot Deaths), 23 St Peter's Square, London W6 9WW. Tel: 01-748-7768

Diabetes
British Diabetic Association, 10 Queen Ann Street, London W1M 0BD

Eczema
National Eczema Society, Tavistock House North, Tavistock Square, London WC1H 95R

Hyperactivity
The Hyperactive Children's Support Group, 59 Meadowside, Angmering, West Sussex
(Enclose SAE + 20p stamps)

Migraine
Migraine Trust, 45 Great Ormond Street, London WC1N 3HD

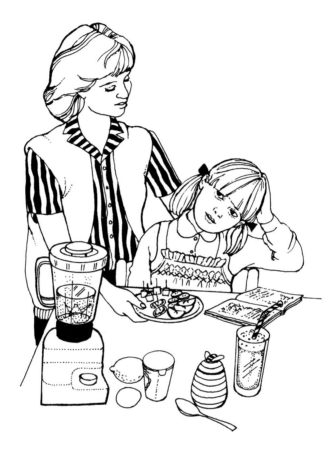

General Index

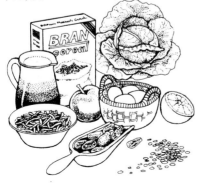

C

U

V

W

X Y Z

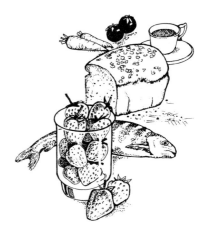

Recipe Index